# Behavioral Approaches to Treating Obesity

2nd edition

*Helping Your Patients Make Changes That Last*

**Birgitta Adolfsson,** PhD
**Marilynn S. Arnold,** MS, RD

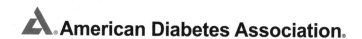
**American Diabetes Association**

*Director, Book Publishing,* Abe Ogden; *Managing Editor,* Greg Guthrie; *Acquisitions Editor,* Victor Van Beuren; *Editor,* Greg Guthrie; *Production Manager,* Melissa Sprott; *Composition,* ADA; *Cover Design,* ADA; *Printer,* Data Reproductions Corporation.

Printed in the United States of America
1 3 5 7 9 10 8 6 4 2

The suggestions and information contained in this publication are generally consistent with the *Clinical Practice Recommendations* and other policies of the American Diabetes Association, but they do not represent the policy or position of the Association or any of its boards or committees. Reasonable steps have been taken to ensure the accuracy of the information presented. However, the American Diabetes Association cannot ensure the safety or efficacy of any product or service described in this publication. Individuals are advised to consult a physician or other appropriate health care professional before undertaking any diet or exercise program or taking any medication referred to in this publication. Professionals must use and apply their own professional judgment, experience, and training and should not rely solely on the information contained in this publication before prescribing any diet, exercise, or medication. The American Diabetes Association—its officers, directors, employees, volunteers, and members—assumes no responsibility or liability for personal or other injury, loss, or damage that may result from the suggestions or information in this publication.

∞ The paper in this publication meets the requirements of the ANSI Standard Z39.48-1992 (permanence of paper).

ADA titles may be purchased for business or promotional use or for special sales. To purchase more than 50 copies of this book at a discount, or for custom editions of this book with your logo, contact the American Diabetes Association at the address below, at booksales@diabetes.org, or by calling 703-299-2046.

American Diabetes Association
1701 North Beauregard Street
Alexandria, Virginia 22311

DOI: 10.2337/9781580404631

**Library of Congress Cataloging-in-Publication Data**

Adolfsson, Birgitta.
  Behavioral approaches to treating obesity : helping your patients make changes that last / Birgitta Adolfsson, Marilynn S. Arnold. -- 2nd ed.
      p. ; cm.
  Includes bibliographical references and index.
  ISBN 978-1-58040-463-1 (alk. paper)
  I. Arnold, Marilynn S. II. American Diabetes Association. III. Title.
  [DNLM: 1. Obesity--prevention & control. 2. Patient Education as Topic--methods. 3. Health Behavior. 4. Life Style. 5. Obesity--psychology. 6. Professional-Patient Relations. WD 210]
  LC classification not assigned
  616.3'98--dc23
                    2011030864

# Contents

# Foreword to the Second Edition

In the past five years, problems related to obesity have grown despite medical, organizational, and environmental improvements designed to offer better treatments and more support. We hope that within the next five years, serious attention and creative problem solving will yield substantial improvement in each of those arenas.

However, serious attention and creative problem solving is also required of individuals who seek long-term weight reduction and improved health. This book continues to offer suggestions for teaching patients *how to solve problems*, a most powerful gift.

For this second edition, we are indebted to our astute reviewers and the supportive ADA editorial staff for guiding us through the revision process.

Birgitta Adolfsson, PhD
Marilynn S. Arnold, MS, RD
March 2011

# Acknowledgments

Although we've never met in person, we chose to author this book together because we were linked by colleagues who have been powerful mentors for each of us. The personal and professional lives of Bob Anderson, Marti Funnell, and the late Anita Carlson personify the philosophical foundation of this book. Many people have read about their philosophy of care, but experiencing firsthand the kind of relationship they advocate confirms the power of everything they have written. Our core agreement with our colleagues' approach to patient-provider relationships made it often possible to understand each other's intent while we worked on the language needed to describe it to others.

To our other colleagues working with the problem-solving model, collaborative care, and lifestyle change, we thank Barbara Anderson, Ingalena Andersson, Betty Brackenridge, Elisabeth Grimholm, and Birgit Hannikainen.

To our supportive and patient friends, Wally Arnold, Nan Bidlack, Per Eriksson, Joan Goodwin, Ingrid Linde, Gudrun Persson, Margareta Lundgren, Margit Lundqvist, Anna-Lena and Loffe Undén Elofsson, and Ulla Vedda, we also owe a heartfelt acknowledgment.

To Bernt Lindahl and Chris Wallin, for their interest in obesity treatment and their support for working with the problem-solving model and lifestyle change, we thank them for their insight.

We thank our colleagues with the Obesity Unit and Clinic of Metabolism and Endocrinology at the Karolinska University Hospital, Stockholm, and with the Michigan Diabetes Research and Training Center at the University of Michigan, Ann Arbor.

We are indebted to the wisdom of Robin Nwankwo, Betty Brackenridge, and Rachel Trevathon, dietitians whose professional practice remains consistent with their understanding that prefabricated solutions rarely fit anyone's personal food habits or style.

Betty Brackenridge is owed further thanks, as is Chris Swensen. They documented that significant improvement in outcome measures are possible when patients receive the information and support they need to make informed decisions about their care.

This book would not exist were it not for the interest, questions, and feedback provided by students, health care providers, and other participants in seminars, lectures, and workshops.

Acknowledgment must be given to all those who helped us appreciate that living with a chronic disease is difficult, that there is always more to the story than is told, and that our professional challenge is to control our comments, not their behavior.

For our colleagues, family, friends, and patients who have demonstrated with their lives the effectiveness of the problem-solving model, who make it clear that they are in charge of their lives, and who demonstrated the power of personal goals in propelling change, we thank them for their inspiration.

To Stig Lundquist, whose feedback on the first version of the manuscript was invaluable, and to our reviewers, who shared their time, effort, expertise, insight, and suggestions to improve the text, we owe a gracious thanks.

To Victor Van Beuren, Christine Charlip, Greg Guthrie, Abe Ogden, and others at the American Diabetes Association, we owe our thanks for their support of the idea of this book and for guiding it through to this finished product.

Finally, we must acknowledge and dedicate this book to our patients, for whom this book is written. Without their trust, courage, and willingness to share their stories, we would not be where we are today in the realm of supporting behavior change. We must thank our patients for the privilege of watching resistance to behavior change dissolve when they realized that no one was pushing.

Birgitta Adolfsson, PhD
Marilynn S. Arnold, MS, RD, LD, CDE
February 2006

# Why This Book?

"Watch your weight." How many of you have told a patient that at one time or another? "Your blood sugar is just a little bit out of range, but if you watch your weight, it will be okay." "Your blood pressure should be fine if you just watch your weight." "You know your knee wouldn't bother you so much if you would just watch your weight."

But what does it mean to "watch your weight"? Is it handing out a flyer with a 1,500-calorie meal plan, recommending the South Beach Diet, or suggesting joining Weight Watchers? These suggestions provide advice that is a bit more specific. Many obese people hear admonitions to consume no sweets, no alcohol, no potatoes, and little fat, but have no clue as to what they should eat. What is helpful? What does no harm?

The recent increase in obesity is a serious global problem, but it is not anyone's fault any more than is a flu epidemic. It is a problem we must solve. We can't choose the effectiveness of our metabolism. We also didn't choose to live in the 21st century, when food that could fill up a polar bear is conveniently available year-round and when desk jobs are prevalent. Although we are not responsible for all of these problems, we can decide how to respond to the situation in which we find ourselves.

Changing how we respond means changing our lifestyle. It means changing the usual behavior patterns (of eating and activity) for those who want to lose weight. It may also mean changing the behavior patterns of those professionals who are interested in helping others lose weight. Usual health care responds well when treating severe and short-term problems (such as the flu or a broken leg), but it is often at a disadvantage when advocating lifestyle change. This is because overweight and obesity are chronic rather than acute conditions and the direct health consequences arise over time. When a person is ill or has a broken leg, the consequences are immediate and felt. Similarly, the solutions are clear cut and directive (e.g., take this medicine, immobilize the leg). People with a chronic condition face the challenge of adjusting to that condition over the long term. They can benefit from the information and support of their health care providers, but effective treatment requires their investment in making changes in the way they live.

Therefore, to support lifestyle change, we must ask ourselves how lifestyle change actually happens. Here are just some thoughts for a discussion on facilitating change.

- Can health care providers diagnose and treat another person's lifestyle?
- Who owns the problem?
- Who lives with the consequences?
- Who does most of the work to solve the problem?
- Where do people get help?
- What kind of help is useful?

Obesity is a chronic condition. Health care planners ascribe a different health care model or paradigm for treating those problems that evolve slowly over time. Chronic conditions cannot be resolved with pills, diets, support groups, counseling, or supplements. The person with the condition must participate. Any or all of the above tools and strategies may prove helpful, but only to the extent that the person with the condition decides to use them.

Assume that a new health care group in town, "The Chronic Care Experiment (TCCE)," approached you about employment. In TCCE, patients are responsible for making all of the decisions about their care, and your role as a health care provider will be to prepare them for that responsibility. This is frequently called the empowerment model for chronic illness, and in such a chronic-care model, you will be a consultant, not the decision maker. Would you decline the position immediately or consider it? How might that job be different from your current one? Would you have to change how you relate to patients or learn new skills?

This book is not a comprehensive obesity text or a new way to lose weight. It is not a bag of tricks and tips to get people to shed pounds. It is an invitation to view the obesity problem from a perspective that we think opens up treatment possibilities. We are a dietitian and psychologist, persuaded by our beloved colleagues, Bob Anderson, Marti Funnell, and the late Anita Carlson, that in chronic care, *patients do make all of the decisions*. From the findings of experts and the teaching of our patients, we offer ideas for applying this philosophy of care to people struggling with obesity.

# Assessing
# the Problem

# Chapter 1

# The Global Challenge of Obesity

*O*besity is a problem. Excess body fat, also known as adipose tissue, is a prominent risk factor for many chronic health problems, including diabetes, heart disease, stroke, cancer, joint problems, and psychosocial stress. Increases in weight drive a similar rise in chronic disease (WHO 2009). Reducing excess fat is a challenge for those who carry it, those who attempt to treat it, and those who pay for its multiple consequences.

We are all likely aware that the rates of obesity have increased dramatically (15 to 34%) in the past 30 years (CDC 2010), despite an ever-expanding array of products, programs, and treatments promoted as remedies. Efforts to reduce the number of people with obesity and to lessen the extent to which they suffer from it present a complex global challenge.

Genetics and environment contribute to obesity, but the rapid increase in obesity rates within the past decade follows a change in human behavior, not a change in genetic makeup (Hill 2006). Today, our unchanged biology, one that has undergone millennia of evolution, survives in an environment in which the pace of change rapidly outstrips the rate of adaptation. It is an environment that in multiple ways supports less activity and invites caloric excess. There is no one way to address the obesity problem, but there are multiple opportunities to reshape our physical environment and adjust our responses to the situation at hand.

In addition to the continuing work of medical science, curbing the obesity explosion poses behavior-related challenges at three distinct levels, each of which has a different role and responsibility in addressing this issue.

1. *To the individual*, who assumes responsibility for his or her self-care decisions.
2. *To the health care system*, which informs and supports individual efforts to make sustainable dietary and activity lifestyle changes.
3. *To society*, which promotes an environment that increases access to **nutrient-dense** food and physical environments that invite activity.

This book is about the second challenge. How do health care professionals interact with patients in a way that supports each individual's innate interest in their own well-being?

# Chapter 2

# The Burden on Society

## Increasing Prevalence

Obesity rates are climbing, not just in the U.S. but also in more and more countries around the world. Figure 1 (page 7) shows the prevalence of obesity around the world (WHO 2000, WHO 2010[a]). The current number of obese Americans is the highest ever recorded. The escalating health risks due to obesity increase the prevalence of chronic disease and health care costs around the world.

Obesity is defined as abnormal and excessive fat accumulation that may impair health (WHO 2009). To assess the health risks of obesity, clinicians use body mass index (BMI), a measure of weight compared with height. BMI is an imperfect tool, but provides a more useful measure of total body fat than weight alone. BMI risk levels are based on the association between BMI and morbidity/mortality for adults over 20 years of age and are the same for both sexes. According to BMI categories, all people with a BMI of 25 kg/m$^2$ or greater are considered overweight. Overweight subcategories are pre-obese for a BMI of 25–29.9 kg/m$^2$ and clinically obese for a BMI $\geq$30 kg/m$^2$ (CDC 2010). As a general estimate of body fat, BMI is helpful for comparing populations, but consideration of factors such as age (older adults lose muscle and gain fat), fitness level (athletes have more muscle), and genetic variation (cutoff points are lower in Asian populations) may modify risk points for individuals.

Based on these criteria, The National Health and Nutrition Examination Survey (NHANES) 2007–2008 (Ogden 2010) reveals that in the U.S.

- 68% of adults older than 20 years are overweight, and 34% of that population is obese
- More men (72%) than women (64%) are overweight, but more women (36%) than men (32%) are obese
- Obesity rates are higher in minority populations, especially among women: 50% of non-Hispanic blacks, 43% of all Hispanics, and 33% of non-Hispanic white females are obese
- Overall, 6% of people are extremely obese, with a BMI ≥40 kg/m²

Data from the NHANES surveys (1976–1980 and 2003–2006) show that the prevalence of obesity has increased for children from 5.0% to over 17% during that period (CDC 2010).

BMI in childhood correlates significantly with BMI in adulthood (Ferraro 2003, Zhao 2011). Young people who are already obese at age 10–15 years are fast becoming the adults who continue to gain weight at the rate of 1.8–2.0 pounds per year between 20 and 40 years of age (Pi-Sunyer 2005). The problems associated with obesity are poised to worsen. Figure 1, opposite, helps show how obesity is becoming a worsening global problem.

# Escalating Burden

As obesity rates rise, the negative consequences of the condition increase. The costs of obesity to society include impaired physical health, impaired mental well-being, and diverted financial resources.

# Impaired Physical Health

Obese persons generally experience more health and mobility problems than do nonobese persons (CDC 2001, Adolfsson 2004). Although not everyone who is obese experiences more health problems than their leaner counterparts (NHLBI 2000), obesity does increase the risk for impaired well-being and for several major diseases.

## Figure 1—Global weight increases, 1991 and most recent available

Key
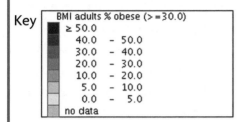

Caveat: The national BMI data displayed in this map are empirical and have been verified that they apply internationally recommended BMI cut-off points. However, it is important to note that the data presented are not directly comparable since they vary in terms of sampling procedures, age ranges, and the year(s) of data collection.

### BMI adults % obese (>=30.0), 1991

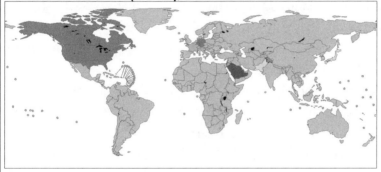

### BMI adults % obese (>=30.0), Most recent

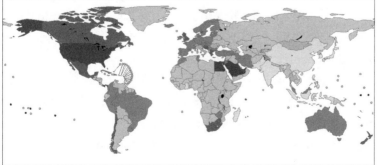

From the WHO Global Database on Body Mass Index. Reprinted with permission from WHO. Available from http://apps.who.int/bmi/index.jsp. Last accessed 13 October 2011.

The link between excess body fat and type 2 diabetes is especially clear. Despite different measures of fatness and different criteria for diagnosing type 2 diabetes, there is a consistent association between excess weight and type 2 diabetes across differing population groups, supporting the strength of this connection (WHO 2000). Colditz (1990) and Chan (1994) report that as many as 65–75% of the people diagnosed with type 2 diabetes would not have developed the disease if their BMI had remained ≤25 kg/m². As a result, the explosive increase in obesity predicts an associated increase in type 2 diabetes. Some have referred to this link between obesity and diabetes as "diabesity" (Zimmet 2001, Astrup 2000).

Sources agree that the number of children (aged <20 years) diagnosed with type 2 diabetes has increased significantly in the past decade, but no data exist to document the number. Minority adolescents, especially if overweight, are those most likely to have type 2 diabetes. A CDC/NIDDK study, Search for Diabetes in Youth, is collecting data to learn more about the character, treatment, and impact of a diabetes diagnosis on children and youth (Mayer-Davis 2009).

Overweight and obesity now rank as the fifth leading global risk for mortality. In addition, 44% of the diabetes burden, 23% of the ischemic heart disease burden, and 7–41% of certain cancer burdens are attributable to overweight and obesity (WHO 2009). Table 1 outlines additional risks associated with obesity (WHO 2000).

Both an individual's fat distribution (i.e., waist circumference) and amount of fat (i.e., BMI) predict health risks (IDF 2006). Abdominal obesity may predict type 2 diabetes more accurately than overall fatness (Pi-Sunyer 2004). (See chapter 7 for more information.)

In addition to the amount and distribution of fat, there is a cluster of disease risk factors that are particularly important to consider when treating overweight or obese individuals (Kahn 2005).

This constellation of interrelated risk factors is often called the metabolic syndrome, and it is strongly associated with obesity, cardiovascular disease, and diabetes. Indicators of metabolic syndrome include dyslipidemia, elevated glucose, hypertension, abdominal obesity, and insu-

## Table 1—Relative Risk of Health Problems Associated with Obesity

| Greatly Increased (relative risk >3) | Moderately Increased (relative risk 2–3) | Slightly Increased (relative risk 1–2) |
|---|---|---|
| Type 2 diabetes | Coronary heart disease | Cancer (breast cancer in post-menopausal women, endometrial cancer, colon cancer) |
| Gallbladder disease | Hypertension | Reproductive hormone abnormalities |
| Dyslipidemia | Osteoarthritis (knees) | Polycystic ovary syndrome |
| Insulin resistance | Hyperuricemia and gout | Impaired fertility |
| Breathlessness | | Lower-back pain due to obesity |
| Sleep apnea | | Increased risk of anesthesia complications |
| | | Fetal defects associated with maternal obesity |

All relative risk values are approximate. Reprinted with permission from WHO (2000).

lin resistance. In combination, these conditions synergistically increase risk. To help identify and treat the underlying problems, sets of diagnostic criteria have been developed. The American Heart Association and the National Heart, Lung, and Blood Institute updated the widely-used National Cholesterol Education Program (NCEP) Adult Treatment Panel III (ATP III) with minor modifications in 2005. The changes in criteria lower the threshold for diagnosis by

1. lowering the cutoff point for elevated blood glucose, and
2. considering a categorical cut point met with drug therapy as a risk factor (Grundy 2005).

The presence of three or more of the risk factors in Table 2 constitutes a diagnosis of metabolic syndrome.

In 2006, the IDF published a worldwide definition of the metabolic syndrome for use in clinical practice. Criteria differ in requiring waist circumference as one of the three risk factors. IDF also offers ethnic-specific values for waist circumference as follows: Caucasian origin, ≥37 inches (≥94 cm) for men and ≥31.5 inches (≥80 cm) for women; South Asian, Jap-

**Table 2—Diagnostic Criteria for Metabolic Syndrome**

| Measure | Categorical Cut Points |
| --- | --- |
| Fasting serum glucose level | ≥100 mg/dl (5.6 mmol/l)<br>or drug treatment for elevated glucose |
| Blood pressure | ≥130/85 mmHg<br>or drug treatment for elevated hypertension |
| Fasting triglycerides | ≥150 mg/dl (1.7 mmol/l)<br>or drug treatment for elevated triglycerides |
| HDL cholesterol | <40 mg/dl in men (1.03 mmol/l)<br><50 mg/dl in women (1.29 mmol/l)<br>or drug treatment for reduced HDL cholesterol |
| Waist circumference | ≥35 inches in women (88 cm)<br>≥40 inches in men (102 cm) |

Adapted from Grundy (2005).

anese, and Chinese origin, ≥35.5 inches (≥90 cm) for men and ≥31.5 inches (≥80 cm) for women (IDF 2006) (See www.idf.org/metabolic-syndrome for additional details).

# Impaired Mental Well-Being

Societal and individual responses to obesity can impair psychological health, which in turn can perpetuate obesity. Prejudices from an unsupportive social environment and social stigmatization are likely to affect psychological health, employment, housing, and overall quality of life (Link 2001). Stigmatization of and discrimination against obese people have been documented in many areas of life, including employment, education, and health care (Puhl 2009). Furthermore, negative attitudes toward obesity by health care professionals can act as a barrier in clinical practice (Teixeira 2010).

Common negative stereotypes attributed to people who are obese include lack of willpower, laziness, ugliness, weak will, emotional and moral instability, as well as being responsible for or to blame for one's weight (Crossow 2001, Friedman 2005, Puhl 2009). The risk for such prevalent negative social messages arises because of the ease with which such attitudes can be internalized; thus, an obese individual may perceive these messages as realistic descriptions of him- or herself (Bacon 2001, Rogge 2004). In response, obese individuals, and those of average weight who feel overweight or obese, may place unnecessary restrictions on important aspects of their lives, such as going to school, changing jobs, buying stylish clothes, dating, enjoying a sexual relationship, and seeking medical care (Robinson 1996).

Women (including those who seek standard treatment as well as more drastic weight-reduction methods, such as surgery) report impaired mental well-being more often than do men or those who do not seek treatment for obesity (Kolotkin 2002). There is an association between a history of weight fluctuation and impaired well-being regardless of body weight (Foreyt 1995).

Impaired mental well-being can precipitate excessive eating as a way of coping with feelings of anxiety, sorrow, and sadness, and thus contribute to obesity (Adolfsson 2002). Excessive eating could also be a coping strategy to deal with obesity-induced stigma (Puhl 2003).

## Growing Economic Burden

As the prevalence of obesity increases, so does the cost of caring for its consequences (Stern 2005). Multiple authors present figures to illustrate the enormous cost of obesity to the health care system, employers, employees, the obese, and the general public.

In 2009, reported annual obesity costs to the health care system range from $147 billion (Finklestein 2010) to $228 billion (Englehard 2009). Because the consequences of obesity are most evident as people age, Medicare/Medicaid pays 50% of this cost (Barkin 2010). Obese employees are more expensive (higher insurance rates) and less productive (Finklestein 2010). Research shows obese employees earn less (Barkin 2010) and pay 42% more for health care than persons of normal weight (Weight-control Information Network 2010). Even nonobese workers pay higher premiums to help cover medical costs of their heavier colleagues (Engle-hard 2009).

As young people gain weight at an increasing rate, their futures, individually and corporately, will be increasingly limited by missed opportunities and by the resources spent to cope with the consequences of obesity. Obese people are often judged less capable and are less often chosen to join a group or perform a job. Physical mobility may limit activities, and health problems reduce available time and money.

WHO and the World Bank recognize that diet-related problems, such as obesity, type 2 diabetes, cardiovascular disease, hypertension, stroke, and various forms of cancer, significantly contribute to disability and premature death in both developing and newly developed countries. Such health problems are overwhelming budgets and absorbing funds from other more traditional public health concerns, such as malnutrition and infectious disease, and placing additional burdens on already overtaxed national health budgets. Obesity is one of the principal contributors to noncommunicable diseases. Given this impaired physical health and its associated economic burden on individuals and societies as a whole, obesity is clearly a risk factor that warrants global attention.

# A Complex Mix of Factors

## Physiological Factors

There are many causes for excess weight. However, genetic makeup clearly contributes to the tendency to gain weight. The gene pool influences body shape, adiposity, and susceptibility to disease. In Maffeis' (2000) review of the literature, he reports that inheritance is responsible for 25–40% of the interindividual differences in adiposity. In 2005, Lyon and Hirschhorn estimated that 30–70% of the variation in obesity within a given population is the result of heredity (Lyon 2005). In most cases, environment greatly influences the expression of genetic material, making parental obesity an important risk factor for obesity in children. Of those who become obese as adolescents, 70% grow up to become obese adults (Zhao 2011). Science is working to uncover the many physiological pathways that influence body weight and to identify ways to interrupt or influence those biological pathways (Zhao 2009).

Medications can also contribute to weight gain. For example, steroids and most antidepressants stimulate hunger. Though such medications are helpful to treat the condition for which they are prescribed, it seems only fair that these side effects be explained and discussed, especially with the patient who is already overweight, before prescribing them.

Changing lifestyle can modify inherited risks, but to what extent? Patients come from different genetic backgrounds and have to play the hand that they are dealt. Therefore, the care providers may find it difficult to assess or appreciate the strength of the biological forces pulling some-one toward food. Notice how patients describe their experience with a food-related problem. It is in this context that they must solve problems.

Over time, science will create more effective treatments for obesity, but lifestyle modification will continue to provide the greatest influence on both health and body weight. Lifestyle refers to the myriad choices that individuals make; those decisions that reflect their personal prefer-ences and shape their daily routines. Lifestyle includes what, where, when, and how much one eats, what clothes the individual chooses to wear, the environment in which one lives and works, social relationships (e.g., family, work, friends), and personal hobbies. Most groups consider our modern lifestyle, particularly sedentary lifestyle and the influence of westernization, to be the cause of worldwide increases in overweight and obesity over the last few decades (WHO 2000).

With high-caloric food, large portions, and snack foods readily avail-able, daily energy intake easily exceeds expenditure. The same genotype expresses itself differently in a hunter-gatherer society than in our soci-ety of computers and fast food. In 2011, the mismatch of our biological makeup and our convenience-driven environment has created a problem to solve. Part of the solution will be to redesign our environment.

# Environmental Factors

Society has created an environment that nurtures obesity. Weight gain is a natural byproduct of modern convenience. There are countless culprits in our modern world: large food portions, desk jobs, remote controls, computer games, machines that do physical work for us, urban sprawl, snack dispensers, elevators, hard-to-find staircases, car culture, clever commercials, fast food, frozen meals, and so on. Individually, any single one of these isn't going to make a population overweight, but when com-bined, these conveniences have reduced the activity levels and increased the caloric intake of an unsuspecting public.

Several new collaborations of local communities, private industry, service organizations, and national government are working to create environments that support physical activity and healthy eating. Resources for individuals and groups of all ages include: the President's Council on Fitness, Sports & Nutrition (www.fitness.gov); Let's Move! (www.letsmove. gov); Shaping America's Youth (www.shapingamericasyouth.org); Small Steps (www.smallstep.gov); Healthy Kids, Healthy Communities (www. healthykidshealthycommunities.org); and a number of state-specific plans.

It is possible to plan environments in which residents can increase activity without thinking about it too much. Environments that support activity could include safe parks and biking trails near homes, building layouts that encourage the use of stairs, and walking (or pedestrian) malls. Several organizations and numerous websites offer information about how to build communities that encourage walking and biking. Among them are the Partnership for a Walkable America (PWA) (www.walkableamerica.org), the Pedestrian and Bicycle Information Center (PBIC) (www.pedbikeinfo.org), and International Walk to School (www.iwalktoschool.org). Information alone will not guarantee behavior change, but by offering environmental support, communities can encourage healthy living by making better choices easier.

Modifying lifestyle is changing usual routines. Change requires time as well as effort. Specifically, to accomplish a lifestyle change, someone must make time for it in his or her usual schedule. Consider two women equally motivated to incorporate a 30-minute walking session three days a week into their lifestyles. The first woman drives to her gym for a 30-minute walk around an indoor track, a drive that takes 15 minutes each way. By the time she's done, she's spent at least 60 minutes on her "exercise session." The second woman lives in a neighborhood where she can simply step out her front door and walk for 30 minutes. Which woman is more likely to stick with her exercise routine and actually increase the number of days she works out in the future?

Hill (2006) proposes that personal responsibility that can be supported by even small changes in the environment offers the most realistic hope for progress.

# Lifestyle

Regardless of genetic background or the medical treatments used, lifestyle choices about food and activity influence body weight. There are multiple physiological pathways in the human species that influence energy balance, and there are even more behavior patterns that influence energy balance in individuals. To make the task of supporting lifestyle change even more difficult, the mechanisms that drive behavior patterns are often not evident and more or less invisible to the person with the behavior. We hope that the difficulty in facilitating behavior change will not dissuade us from pursuing it as a viable (and effective) treatment option. If someone enters a clinic with an infection, do we just treat it or do we look for what is causing the infection? We look for the source of the problem. It is at least as important to look for the source of problematic behavior patterns before considering treatment options.

There are many reasons that prompt people to eat more than they need. Eating more than the body requires is "excessive eating" whether the food portions are large or the caloric content is high. For most people, an appropriate intake at 20 years of age becomes excessive at 40 due to changes in physical activity. Today, hunger is rarely the only reason for eating. Frequently, people eat because they are prompted by habit, because they feel pressured by social circumstances, or because they use it as a way to cope with discomfort.

An iceberg is a useful metaphor to describe the factors that influence obesity (see Fig. 2). We often only interact with the tip of the obesity iceberg—its physical components. Below the waterline are the true obstacles, the behavioral and genetic factors that drive obesity. We are able to make effective, sustained change at the tip of this iceberg if we can trace and address the underlying factors. Health care providers have the opportunity to help patients identify, address, and change the behavioral patterns that encourage excessive eating. The following sections describe reasons obese people report for accumulating excess pounds.

---

**Figure 2—The Iceberg**

BMI
Energy intake
Physical activity
Waist circumference

---

Reasons for excessive eating
Support from significant others
Motivation for lifestyle change
Reasons for limited physical activity
Expectations of the weight-reduction process
Hope • Energy • Future dreams • Stress/balance in life
Self-efficacy • Locus of control • Readiness for change
Emotional and social consequences of lifestyle change
Self-rated health • Social and mental well-being • Physical health • Lifestyle
Expectations of life with a normal BMI • Sexual matters • Socioeconomic situation

---

# Food Habits

Daily food habits often contribute to excessive eating and obesity. Much like a person's genetic makeup, dietary patterns can be passed on from one generation to the next. Children who grow up with high-fat meals, routine snacking in front of the TV, and a well-stocked cookie jar are likely to continue those habits in their own homes, thus perpetuating excess weight regardless of genetics. Habits such as skipping meals, eating while driving, eating take-out meals, and drinking high-calorie beverages can all easily develop in response to tight schedules, family demands, fatigue, poor planning, or social pressure. Awareness, information, and support can help committed individuals change these habits. However, cravings complicate this process.

# Cravings

One of the most common weight-loss questions is why is it so hard to stick with healthy behaviors, even when we know exactly how to eat well and know when we make poor choices? Eating is often affiliated with feelings and needs rather than with what we know to be healthy habits. When excessive eating satisfies underlying needs, those needs must be addressed during weight-reduction treatment or they will obstruct weight loss and interfere with sustained efforts to lose weight.

Figure 3 organizes motives for excessive eating from the iceberg (Fig. 2), similar to Maslow's motivational hierarchy of needs, where a need motivates behavior (Maslow 1968).

Craving, which often leads to excessive eating, is associated with "faulty" hunger awareness, which arises from different biological and psychosocial needs. The biological function of eating—to provide energy for

---

**Figure 3—Excessive Eating and Maslow's Motivational Hierarchy**

5. **Self-Actualization** needs

*seeking personal growth and realizing*
*personal potential*

try new dishes and diets

4. **Appreciation** needs

*prestige and achievement*

eating special food or visiting special restaurants
for some ego reason

3. **Social** needs

*eating brings people together*

2. **Safety** needs

*protection from starvation*

Thousands of years ago, when food was scarce and the risk of starvation a real threat, the ability to store fat saved lives. Although we live in a mainly prosperous society, this mechanism still affects our behavior.

1. **Physiological** needs

*eat to survive*

life—has changed. We expect food to satisfy other human needs. People eat to build a sense of security, affinity, or self-actualization. Thus, to alter the reasons for excessive eating, an obese or overweight person has to discover what function excessive eating serves. There may be a way to make these cravings unnecessary or to create a sense of satisfaction with something other than eating. Emotional reasons for cravings sometimes overlap. The following categories of cravings are arbitrary, but may be helpful in identifying possible sources of cravings. You can find practical approaches to helping the patient solve these issues in chapter 17.

## Stress

Many people eat in response to stress. According to the psychological definition, stress arises from an imbalance between a person's perceived resources and perceived demands (Lazarus 1984). People look for coping skills that help them adapt to and manage that imbalance and may respond to stress with active or passive coping strategies (de Ridder 1997).

Henry (1977) describes active, problem-focused coping as a "fight-or-flight" strategy and passive coping as a "defeat reaction" or loss of control. Eating for comfort is a passive coping strategy (Popkess-Vawter 1998). Reports suggest that these cravings are due to the energizing power of sweets and the calming effect of fats (Wells 1998). Some evidence points to a relationship between the passive coping style and obesity (Hörchner 2002) and with the release of the cortisol hormone (Bob 2008), which is associated with central obesity, type 2 diabetes, and other components of the metabolic syndrome (Ljung 2001, Phillips 2010).

Research shows that obese people use passive coping more often than active, problem-focused coping (Rydén 2003). Hunger has been associated with feelings of hopelessness (Chilton 2007). Eating may offer a way to escape problems that are perceived as too difficult or impossible to solve (Popkess-Vawter 1998). Obese women particularly describe eating as a way to feel better in stressful situations (Laitinen 2002). Due to the significant association between passive coping and central obesity, some researchers interpret abdominal fat as an indicator of hopelessness (Björntorp 1999).

Symptoms of stress can be physiological and psychological. If a person has coped with stress through excessive eating and then stops that eating without addressing the initiating stressors, other stress symptoms may emerge. Feelings of anger, irritation, isolation, and depression, along with impaired memory and concentration, sleep disturbance, palpitations of the heart, hypertension, and tensed muscles could be symptoms of stress overload.

Chronic stress affects the hippocampus, the brain structure that provides information on how the environment is organized (Sapolsky 1996). Thus, stress may fragment and distort a person's assessment of their environment and impair their learning and memory (Ivy 2010). This phenomenon has many implications for health care providers. For example, receiving a diagnosis of diabetes or any other medical problem is usually traumatic and stressful. Initially, patients may have difficulty understanding and assimilating medical or dietary recommendations, because the world with which they must interact has become radically different. Some time and/or help to adjust to the diagnosis may reduce the stress and therefore increase the patient's ability to understand, accept, and act on the information that is provided. Patients, seen in clinical practice, report that after learning new coping strategies for stress, it becomes much easier to follow dietary recommendations.

## Sensitivity to Stimuli and Avoiding Monotony

Obese people are more inclined to act impulsively, avoid monotony, and respond to external cues, such as the sight or availability of food, than are people of normal weight (Rydén 2004). Instead of keeping up with dietary routines, the person easily gives in to satisfy a craving. A conflict between enjoying instant rewards and achieving long-term results develops. Stress overload sometimes decreases the threshold for responding to external cues for eating. The media and "soap operas" often portray life

*back of sleep ⟹ ↑level of cortisol ⟹ obesity*

to be a matter of passion or pain. On the contrary, much of life consists of following routines and is often a rather monotonous story, quite unlike television drama. Establishing healthy dietary habits is especially helpful for people with low impulse tolerance.

## Unsatisfactory Sleep and Fatigue

Excessive eating and obesity have been associated with disturbed or unsatisfactory sleep (Vardar 2004, Patel 2004). Many obese people suffer from sleep apnea (WHO 2009), and abdominal obesity has been strongly associated with sleep disturbances. Lack of sleep has been associated with increased levels of cortisol (Chaput 2010), and increased cortisol levels have been associated with abdominal obesity (Zinn 2010).

The literature also reports a social prejudice, even among health care personnel, against obese people as lazy and lacking willpower (Puhl 2009). In order to fight this prejudice, obese people sometimes feel the need to work harder and longer than normal-weight people. Some may unconsciously believe that excessive eating will give them strength, and they ignore sensations of fatigue or lack of energy while working harder. This trend, obviously, leads to more fatigue and can ultimately result in further weight gain.

## Inability to Differentiate Between Physical and Emotional Sensations

People who grew up in an environment where neither physical nor emotional needs were met may be unable to accurately differentiate among various unpleasant physiological and emotional states (Bruch 1973, Rydén 2004). These people may overeat in response to virtually any internal arousal state. They interpret emotional distress as hunger and/or craving.

## Anxiety and Other Painful Feelings

Anxiety is a general uneasiness in which someone feels a sense of danger or of an impending catastrophe. The intensity can vary. Psychological defenses protect against anxiety (Freud 1979). Some people use excessive eating as a defense against anxiety (Rydén 2004, Mills 1994, Slochower 1980, 1981). Eating and the resulting feelings of physical satisfaction can also soothe and comfort other feelings, such as anger, depressed mood, sorrow, shame, guilt, and loneliness (Adolfsson 2002, Wilson 2003, Poston 2000, Bulik 2007).

## Sexual Issues

Sexual satisfaction and intimacy are important parts of life that contribute to physical and emotional well-being. Physical satisfaction that is achieved from eating can balance various forms of distress: sex anxiety, anger, sadness, sorrow, and loneliness (Cooper 1986, McDougall 1989, Rydén 2004). Oxytocin is a "calmness hormone," released by massage, sexual arousal, and orgasm as well as by the consumption of fat (Carmichael 1987, Uuvnäs Moberg 1999). Some people achieve a feeling of balance and peace through intimate relationships that provide sexual satisfaction and support in times of distress. Others find this balance and peace through the consumption of fat.

Changes in behavior and/or in weight may impact relationships. Jeffery (2002) reports an association between weight change and the relationships between spouses. Sometimes the connection between obesity and sexuality is used to stabilize an unhealthy relationship, so that partners perceive weight changes as a threat to the relationship as they know it. If a formerly obese partner becomes more sexually active after weight reduction, it disturbs the status quo and may cause relationship problems (Marshall 1977). If sexual intimacy has previously provoked anxiety or trauma, some people learn to depend on their obesity to avoid sexually intimate situations (Wiederman 1999). King (1996) reports that obese victims of sexual abuse experience more difficulties losing weight than those who were not sexually abused, unless they receive treatment for their trauma. Because the long-term effects of sexual abuse can interfere with obesity treatment, a history of sexual abuse may be an important pretreatment variable to consider (Feldman 2007).

## Interruption of Group Expectations

Eating has a social function (Jastran 2009). Meals often bring people together. Food preferences and eating and meal habits may express belonging in a social network. Social gatherings and social traditions are often centered on shared meals, where eating can function as a "social glue" and hide interpersonal discomfort. If a person's food choices differ from the group's usual menu, then that "glue" may deteriorate. Figure 4 illustrates how a change in one member of a group will often require change for the other members of the group.

A family is a type of system in which the members know what to

**Figure 4—Symbolic Illustration of How Change in One Area Causes Change in Another**

If one person (white piece) changes, those close to him or her are also forced to change. This compounds the difficulty of lifestyle change because not only must an individual work at making the behavior change a lifestyle habit, but he or she must also deal with the responses of others to that change.

Before change

After change

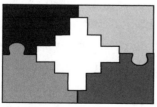
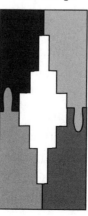

expect from each other. If one family member makes a lifestyle change, the family system changes, which affects the other members in that system. When one member threatens the status quo, the group's initial reaction is to make another change, hoping to reestablish homeostasis. This reactive manipulation may include flattery, aggression, nagging, threats, or even rejection from the group. One client reported a friend telling her directly that their friendship was over if the client lost weight. Though logic questions the quality of these relationships, rejection is not a price that everybody is willing or ready to pay. Thus, it is important to address reactions and problems that might arise if the homeostasis in a social system is disturbed. Otherwise, family members', friends', or colleagues' responses may block behavior change efforts (Papero 1990). A systems approach that addresses the deleterious impact of psychosocial stressors on health and lifestyle issues would help participants achieve the greatest benefits from lifestyle change activities (Porter 2010).

## Physical Activity

Reduced physical activity increases risks for metabolic syndrome (Eckel 2005, Pritchett 2005). As the world has entered the 21st century, our desire for convenience, comfort, and speed has continued to influence decisions that affect our everyday lives, including how we prepare food (i.e., someone else does it) and design buildings (elevators are more convenient than stairs). But this ideological shift has even changed the way we view other less obvious lifestyle habits, such as how we clean (convenient devices never require scrubbing or any sweat), how we interact with our environment (power tools and fancy motorized kitchen utensils remove the need for working hard), and how we relax (remote controls clutter coffee tables like magazines did in years past). Driving through a fast food restaurant after working late and eating in front of the television has become normal behavior.

The 2008 Physical Activity Guidelines for Americans (CDC 2011[b]) recommend 150 minutes of moderate-intensity (brisk walk) aerobic

activity, 75 minutes of vigorous-intensity aerobic activity, or an equiva-
lent mix of the two each week. The guidelines also recommend muscle-
strengthening activities on two or more days a week that work all major
muscle groups (legs, hips, back, abdomen, chest, shoulders, and arms).
Recommendations suggest that everyone, including older adults, benefit
from both aerobic and muscle-strengthening activity geared to their fitness level.

The American College of Sports Medicine (Donnelly 2009) reports
that some individuals require even more exercise (150–250 minutes per
week of moderate-intensity physical activity) just to prevent weight gain.
If our normal routine of work and/or play does not regularly include this
amount of activity, we must either intentionally commit to an exercise
routine or live with the bulges that store this unspent energy. Of adults
over 19 years of age, an average of 46% met the 2008 recommendations
for aerobic exercise and 21% met both aerobic and muscle-strengthening
recommendations in 2010. Participation in physical activity was lower
than this among women, older adults, and minorities (CDC/NCHS 2011).

# Chapter 4

# Treatment Options

As the rate of obesity increases, so has our appreciation that this condition is complex. The age-old approach to weight loss—calories consumed must be balanced against calories expended—is not incorrect but is far from complete. Genetic susceptibility and environmental encouragement have joined forces to boost consumption and minimize activity, accelerating the incidence and consequences of excess body weight. Several tools, supported by medical research, are available for fighting excess weight. However, tools alone assist but do not solve the problem. Sustainable weight loss still requires that the number of calories out surpasses the number of calories in. To accomplish this, we offer information and support on how to change, teach the basics of meal planning, and invite everyone to move more and sit less. If these patient-driven activities are insufficient, drug therapy and bariatric surgery may be appropriate adjuncts.

WHO (2007) and NHLBI (2010) describe methods that address caloric balance. The stated goal is to reduce energy intake so that it is lower than calories burned during the weight-loss phase and to rebalance caloric intake to match calorie expenditure during the weight-maintenance phase. Successful long-term weight loss has been defined as an intentional 10% weight reduction from baseline that is maintained for one year (Wing 2005). To reduce calories eaten or to increase calories burned requires change.

# Lifestyle Change

Behavioral treatment is an essential component of any credible obesity treatment program (Berkel 2005, Foster 2004). Besides addressing the explicit problem behavior, behavioral treatment also addresses the ideas and emotions associated with having and changing behavior (Foster 2005). The primary targets for lifestyle change are eating habits and physical activity levels. However, changing behavior is, by itself, a skill that must be learned. Learning how to change is akin to learning how to learn. Once established, those skills offer the individual the power to keep changing and learning in the future. Successfully making changes is much more likely if people experience support for their efforts as well as guidance. Because obesity is a chronic condition, gaining skill and confidence in how to change behavior is vital to sustained weight loss.

## The Core Features of Behavioral Treatment

- *Observation.* Self-monitor eating habits and physical activity.
- *Stimulus control.* Identify and limit exposure to cues that prompt overeating.
- *Cognitive restructuring.* Identify and modify unrealistic goals and inaccurate beliefs about weight regulation.
- *Social support.* Identify others who can help support your behavior change efforts.
- *Problem solving.* Address issues related to eating and physical activity.
- *Relapse prevention.* Engage in maintenance of the achieved weight loss. Reevaluate setbacks and view these as learning experiences rather than failures.

Behavioral treatment can also include stress management (NHLBI 1998) and support for balanced and flexible food choices instead of structured diets as a means to improving nutrition (WHO 2000).

# Meal Planning

"Meal planning" replaces the term "diet" and refers to the professionally recommended plan for improving someone's dietary intake. Such plans are based on portion sizes, nutrient composition, and food distribution intakes that are likely to facilitate weight control. However, the actual meal plan as devised with a patient may only identify specific actions to help move the usual eating pattern toward a recommended one. Examples may be to add an apple to lunch, include a late afternoon snack, and/or switch from soft drinks to tea or water. Many patients benefit from more structure (calculated meal plans, recipes, prepared food) or simplified meals (a week of menus), especially in the beginning. People often have much to learn about how to select and prepare food. The work we do with a patient to devise an eating strategy is called meal planning.

Meal planning is an essential component of all weight-management strategies. A plan that somehow lowers caloric intake is typically necessary for weight loss, but this does not necessarily mean that an individual will always need to consume a smaller amount (volume) of food or actually count calories. Plans can change. The goal, as always, is to devise a meal plan that fits the individual who plans to use it.

---

## Core Considerations for Building Meal Plans

*Renee*

- Space food intake to fuel energy needs and avoid excess hunger
- Limit portion size and frequent snacking
- Choose foods that supply nutrients, which contribute to health by:
  - ◆ Eating a variety of foods from all of the food groups
  - ◆ Emphasizing high-fiber plant food: whole grains, fruits, vegetables, cooked dried beans, nuts, seeds, etc.
  - ◆ Choosing lean protein
  - ◆ Minimizing saturated and/or trans fat intake
- Consume adequate non-caloric fluids

*Sources:* USDA/USDHHS 2010, NHLBI 2005

# Physical Activity

According to the 2008 Physical Activity Guidelines for Americans, health improves with at least 150 minutes of aerobic activity and two days of strength training per week. Specifically, guidelines recommend that, for good health, people set as their weekly target 150 minutes (30 minutes for 5 days) of moderate-intensity aerobic activity (i.e., brisk walking) and muscle-strengthening activities on two or more days per week (CDC 2011[b]). Recommendations suggest that everyone benefits from both aerobic and muscle-strengthening activity. This assumes type, intensity, and duration match individual needs. Appropriate exercise may require professional guidance, especially for those with physical limitations / disability.

Additional exercise is probably required to support weight-loss efforts. Moderate-intensity physical activity for 150–250 minutes per week provides modest weight loss, which can be improved with modest (but not severe) diet restrictions. Physical activity greater than 250 minutes per week is more likely to result in clinically significant weight loss (Donnelly 2009). Although resistance training does not significantly enhance weight loss, it does increase loss of fat mass and improves health risks with or without weight loss. Because muscle burns calories, increasing muscle mass increases calorie needs.

There is evidence that ongoing physical activity helps maintain weight loss (Cooper 2001, Hill 2005). Although the amount required varies greatly from person to person, it is likely that as much as or more (>250 minutes per week) physical activity is required to maintain weight loss (CDC 2011[a]). Currently, there is no evidence from randomized controlled trials to document physical activity effectiveness to prevent regain (Donnelly 2009).

Although the impact of exercise on weight loss may be modest, both the International Diabetes Federation (IDF 2010) and the CDC (2011[a]) recommend increased physical activity for weight loss. Exercise as part of a comprehensive weight-loss therapy and weight-maintenance program may decrease body fat and increase lean muscle (U.S. Department of Health and Human Services 2005[a,b]), as well as offering cardiovascular and other health benefits. Unfortunately, the short-term costs of sacrificing free time, physical comfort, and convenience often seem to outweigh the benefits of a more active lifestyle. Nevertheless, increased physical activity makes successful weight loss more likely.

Many formerly obese people testify that establishing regular routines for physical activity was a turning point in maintaining lifestyle changes. Functional impairment and chronic pain are more prevalent among obese people compared with people in other weight groups (WHO 2000, Larsson 2002, Marcus 2004). Support from health care personnel may be necessary for clients to find ways to be physically active without increasing pain. Facilitating access to safe exercise offers special-needs clients a proven tool for weight-loss maintenance and improved health.

# Drug Treatment

For some people, drug therapy for weight loss can be a short-term adjunct to behavior change, meal planning, and activity. Drug treatment may be considered for patients with a BMI $\geq 30$ kg/m$^2$ if treatment with diet, exercise, and behavior change has proven insufficient to reach goals. Drug treatment can also be considered for patients with substantial comorbidities associated with a BMI $\geq 27$ kg/m$^2$ (NIDDK 2007) that have persisted despite improved diet, exercise, and behavior treatment. Although drugs cannot override poor eating habits for sustained weight loss, they can make successful weight loss more attainable and support continued behavior change. Drug therapy can support weight maintenance as well as weight loss.

There have been two types of weight-management drugs. One type targets the gastrointestinal system to inhibit nutrient absorption or cause a feeling of satiety. The other acts on the central nervous system to influence feeding behavior and suppress appetite. For many years there was one available drug for each of these types. The first, orlistat, is now available over-the-counter in a reduced dose and by prescription (FDA 2010[a]).

med ↓ wt → Orlistat → OTC

Late in 2010, the second drug, sibutramine, which acts on the central nervous system, was removed from the market due to increased cardiac risks (FDA 2010[b]). A few months later, the FDA removed a supplement (Fruta Planta) from the market when it was found to contain that same drug (FDA 2011[a]). Before the end of 2010, the FDA also denied approval for two new obesity drugs (Qnexa and Lorcaserin) (Pollack 2010[a,b]) and granted preliminary approval to a third. Providers were hopeful, as the third drug (Contrave) was a combination of two drugs already on the market, but early in 2011, the third drug was sent back for additional testing (FDA 2011[b]).

Given the overwhelming rise in obesity, there is an ever-growing demand for treatment options. Because millions will take a new weight-loss drug and the risks for adverse reactions are high, the FDA seeks evidence that a drug's benefits clearly outweigh the risks before allowing it to reach the market.

To ensure safety and efficacy, WHO, NIH, and others emphasize that these drugs are only for weight management conducted with medical supervision and in combination with behavior change therapy. Weight-loss drugs do not offer successful treatment for those unwilling to make changes.

Keep in mind that medications for other problems may also influence weight-reduction efforts. If extra eating stems from feelings of depression, appropriate treatment for depression may aid weight loss. On the one hand, many antidepressants stimulate hunger and could have the opposite effect.

For people living with diabetes, understanding how diabetes medications impact hunger is the key to managing weight. To regulate blood glucose levels, digested food and insulin must be available in the bloodstream at the same time. Biguanides plus the newer oral medications (DPP-4 inhibitors, incretin mimetics, and antihyperglycemic synthetic analogs) help accomplish this without the risk of providing or stimulating excess insulin.

Excessive or improperly timed insulin or insulin-stimulating oral diabetes medications may stimulate hunger and/or the need for extra snacking to avoid hypoglycemia. Two oral medications stimulate increased insulin production. Sulfonylureas are longer acting and taken once or twice a day. Meglitinides are shorter acting but must be taken 5–30 minutes before each meal. People treated with the longer-acting sulfonylurea are more likely to experience hypoglycemia in the late afternoon if they skip or eat too little for lunch. The trade off is more frequent dosing versus more attention to one's eating schedule.

When treatment with insulin is necessary, understanding the action time of the insulin is essential for coordinating injections with food intake. For example, rapid-acting insulin peaks in 1–2 hours and best matches a balanced meal when taken within 15 minutes of the first bite of food. Among insulin pump users, a common problem is taking extra insulin to lower a high blood glucose level before the insulin already present in the bloodstream has finished working. This often results in hypoglycemia. This experience is usually unpleasant enough that those experiencing it want to feel better right away. There is a strong temptation to treat the hypoglycemia with more food than is needed, setting up a cycle of eating extra food, resulting in hyperglycemia that has to be treated with extra insulin, which leads to more hypoglycemia.

Preventing hypoglycemia does much to limit calorie intake. Treating hypoglycemia appropriately with 15–30 grams of carbohydrate also helps limit calorie intake. Treating hypoglycemia with a fat-containing food (such as peanut butter crackers or a candy bar) adds extra calories, slows the rate of carbohydrate absorption, delays recovery, and often leads to another high glucose reading. For further information about weight issues for those with diabetes, see *Diabetes Nutrition Q & A for Health Professionals* (ADA 2003).

The hunger that accompanies hyperglycemia itself may subside when diabetes is treated. A well-managed plan for blood glucose control makes a major contribution to weight management.

Apart from drug therapy for obesity, monitoring the side effects of other medications can help everyone avoid unnecessary barriers to weight-loss efforts.

# Bariatric Surgery

Bariatric surgery provides another treatment option when dietary, exercise, and behavior change efforts supported by weight-reducing drugs (when available) prove insufficient to reduce health risks.

As the negative consequences of obesity increase and surgical techniques improve, the cost-to-risk ratio has improved, and bariatric surgery has become more common for people whose obesity is a serious health threat. In fact, the number of surgeries increased 10-fold during the six years between 1998 and 2004 (Kulick 2010).

Different surgical methods assist weight loss by reducing stomach size (restricting storage space), by reducing nutrient absorption, and/or by influencing hormones that reduce appetite. By reducing stomach capacity, excess food has nowhere to go, making the consequences of overeating rather unpleasant and reinforcing the habit of eating smaller portions. Surgeries that also reduce absorption result in greater weight loss but also in higher risks for malnutrition.

Guidelines suggest that appropriate patients are those with a BMI $\geq$40 kg/m$^2$ or a BMI $\geq$35 kg/m$^2$ with high-risk, life-threatening comorbid conditions (NIDDK 2009). Although surgical procedures are more expensive and come with higher risks for serious complications, preliminary research supports substantial improvement in comorbidities (Ayman 2010) that reduce overall risk (Picot 2009).

Early in 2011, the FDA lowered the cutoff point for the surgery that uses an adjustable gastric banding system. This device, implanted around the upper part of the stomach, limits the amount of food that can be eaten at one time and is now a treatment option for people with a life-threatening comorbid condition (including diabetes) and a BMI $\geq$30 kg/m$^2$ instead of $\geq$35 kg/m$^2$. People seeking this surgery must also be willing to make major changes to their lifestyle and eating habits. For those without an obesity-related comorbid condition, the BMI cutoff point for this surgery remains $\geq$40 (FDA 2011$^c$).

Successful candidates for bariatric surgery have acceptable operative risks and are motivated, willing to become well informed, and willing to participate in continuing programs that support behavior change. The keys to successful bariatric surgery include changing behavior patterns, accessing support systems, and long-term follow-up (Dowd 2005). More specific recommendations address meal timing, portion control, food quality, and the need for exercise. Note that behavior change, exercise, follow-up, and support are the same ingredients required for success using nonsurgical approaches to weight-loss (Franz 2007).

# Always Behavior Change

Regardless of the approach to weight loss, behavior change is a required component. Whether it addresses changing a habit, such as late-night snacking, changing food choices, or adding more activity, patients lose a familiar daily activity. They give up a piece of themselves and enter unfamiliar territory. Even drug therapy requires some behavior change to be successful; patients must make sure that they take the medication as prescribed. The experience of weighing less—regardless of how it is accomplished—also changes people's perceptions of themselves and the way other people respond to them. The following chapters describe a health care model that supports and encourages patients in their efforts to change and offer practical tools for supporting this model's success.

# Chapter 5

# The Paradigm of Care

*"If you want to build a ship,*
*Don't drum up the people to collect wood and*
*Don't assign them tasks and work,*
*But rather teach them to long for the end-less immensity of the sea."*
—Antoine de Saint-Exupery

## Why Change It?

Obesity is a problem with adverse medical consequences, and lifestyle change is an essential part of the solution. A person living with excess weight must be engaged in and commit to changing his or her habits, and many require help in doing so.

Extensive documentation points to lifestyle as the first line of treatment to address the risk factors of metabolic syndrome (Nonas 2004). WHO states that the worldwide increase in obesity arises from lifestyle issues, such as unhealthy eating habits and decreased physical activity. The American Diabetes Association (ADA) and other experts recommend weight loss and increased physical activity as the safest, most effective, and preferred way to reduce insulin resistance in overweight and obese people. Randomized controlled studies show that even a weight loss of 3–5% of total body weight along with improved eating habits and increased physical activity decreases the prevalence of type 2 diabetes by 30–60% among obese people with impaired glucose tolerance (Knowler 2002, Tuomilehto

2001). Although a 5% loss of initial body weight will yield improvement, further benefits accompany a loss of 10% and may be necessary to achieve measurable benefits in those with an initial BMI >35 kg/m$^2$ (SIGN 2010). Providers look for clinically useful changes, such as lowered blood pressure, improved lipids, and better control of diabetes (NCBI 1998, NICE 2006). Lifestyle changes work, but what does it take to make them work?

Much of our eating is informed by the culture in which we live. Society sends conflicting messages about food, health, and weight issues. Although being slim is valued as attractive and healthy by society, messages from advertising and other media undermine efforts to actually practice healthy behaviors. There is no identified connection between eating and slimness in commercial media. The implicit message seems to be that a person can be slim, yet not think about health. Too often, weight concerns are reduced to cosmetic issues. The end result of the contradictions in media messages is a generally unhealthy attitude toward eating and appearance.

Quick-fix diets lead consumers to visualize unrealistic, instant results and cast doubt on the less dramatic benefits of sustained healthy dietary management. There are many products and programs available that market themselves as solutions to the obesity problem. On the one hand, any diet that results in energy restriction and weight loss improves the metabolic profile of an individual (Sacks 2009). However, on the other hand, weight loss can be a marker of improved lifestyle habits or it can be the result of a short-term restricted diet or disordered eating. This ambiguity makes weight change itself an uncertain measure of progress. If the primary goal in treating obesity is to avoid adverse medical consequences, measures of **changed behaviors will serve as more appropriate markers of progress than pounds lost**. The real measure of success for weight-loss interventions is improved health (Dausch 2001).

Body weight is relatively easy to use to measure the results of change and provides an objective tool with which to measure change and compare individuals to population data. However, reliance on weight change as the only or primary measure of progress keeps the focus on the scale and cannot support long-term behavior change. When people hit a plateau or maintenance stage, weight loss will no longer provide positive reinforcement. This is when the importance of persisting with lifestyle change is crucial.

Facilitating behavior change requires a different approach to health care than the traditional acute care approach to medicine. The standard acute care visit addresses short-term problems with a specific recommendation. The provider makes treatment decisions with little need for input from the staff or the patient. Minimal follow-up is needed.

Obesity is a chronic condition. The Chronic Care Model provides a more effective structure for providing care (and reducing the costs) of chronic disease. This comprehensive model includes community, organizational, and clinical components to support its goals. It also emphasizes patient education, support, and access to resources as essential so that the person living with the problem can become an active participant in his or her own care (Blackburn 2005).

With a chronic disease approach, health care systems have the opportunity to advocate for the treatment of obesity as a complex biological/psychosocial problem that requires the tools of evidence-based medicine. By regularly assessing medical risk factors, offering treatment options based on scientific evidence, and providing long-term follow-up, health care providers may be able to **refocus attention on health rather than weight**. In doing this, the core of a treatment program focuses not on solving the "weight problem," but on "increasing health." Whether or not medications or surgery are included, the overall treatment plan requires behavior change to achieve long-term health goals.

Due to the strong association between cultural influences and obesity (e.g., "be thin, eat what you want, be healthy, but don't do anything about it"), obesity simply cannot be treated with the familiar acute-care model. The habits and lifestyle choices that lead to obesity are closely tied to our modern environment, thus simply prescribing a regimen of physical activity and healthy eating will normally fail. If a patient presents with an infection, we treat with the proper antibiotic. That is the rationale behind the acute-care model. However, what if this patient's infection briefly goes away and then comes back quickly? We begin to search for additional causes of this infection. There may be medical reasons, such as the need for a different antibiotic or the presence of another medical problem that reduces resistance.

Furthermore, the problem could be related to the patient's lifestyle. Did the patient take all of his or her antibiotics? Is he or she susceptible to re-infection because he or she is fatigued from inadequate rest? Is the patient experiencing high stress due to unexpected bills? Is he or she smoking, which reduces resistance to infection? Has the patient experienced increased exposure to bacteria from crowds?

If the provider and patient discuss the problem, they could better identify possible causes. The patient may first require information about what may be a potential cause. If potential sources are identified, then the patient may require help knowing what might be done about them. Ultimately, the patient will have to decide what he or she is willing and able to do to reduce the risk of re-infection.

In the chronic-care model, patients do more than follow instructions. They partner in determining the problem and (because they are the ones making the changes) deciding what changes are worth making. This shift from physician-determined treatment to collaboration between the patient and provider defines the chronic-care model and a behavioral approach. **Such a paradigm shift is necessary for the successful treatment of overweight and obesity in the modern world because (whether we as providers like it or not) the patient with chronic disease provides the majority of his or her own care.**

Antoine de Saint-Exupery captured the essence of this paradigm shift. More explicitly it might read:

*If you want optimal health for your patients*
*Don't overload them with information*
*Don't give them lists of dos and don'ts*
*But help them visualize the possibilities with confidence and*
*    discover the passions that energize their choices.*

# Part II

# Designing Care to Address Obesity

# Chapter 6

# Changing Roles

Collaborative care is one cornerstone of the evolving chronic-care model (Wagner 2001). It implies a change in the traditional acute-care paradigm in regard to the roles and relationships between health care providers and patients (Anderson 2005). In chronic care, decisions about lifestyle change require the participation and input of the person doing the changing. Although health care providers bring their expertise to the planning, the patient is the expert on his or her life. Meal plans and physical activity are not like medications, which are simply taken at the proper time. Behavior change is useless until fully integrated into a person's experience and adapted to individual circumstances. The patient is the individual most able to identify the causes of his or her problem, providing insight that ideally shapes the treatment plan. The patient and provider must become equal partners in a successful collaborative chronic-care model.

The key component of effective chronic-disease management is productive interactions between patient and provider. Productive interaction has implications for the role of the patient, the provider, and the system. It substantially changes the familiar style of the patient-provider relationship practice with "the need to alter reactive acute-care–oriented practice to accommodate the proactive, planned, patient-oriented longitudinal care required" (Glasglow 2001). New roles may be uncomfortable at first, but they are necessary to address the complexity, disability, and ongoing nature of chronic disease (Wagner 2001).

# The Patient's Role

The patient's role is to become an informed and active participant in his or her own care. People who are obese must define the problem as it is relevant to them. Not everyone who is obese considers his or her weight a problem. Until and unless they do, no one can solve the problem.

For example, Sally knew how to eat well but ate more than she needed. She saw her excess weight as purely cosmetic. Considering other life challenges to be more interesting than working on her appearance, she made no attempt to lose weight despite periodic prodding by her physician. When diagnosed with diabetes, her priorities changed. After that, changing her eating and activity habits became a worthwhile investment, and she devoted the time and effort needed to improve glycemic control.

Not everyone will be able to define and solve their weight problem as independently as Sally did, but if the patient cannot clearly define the problem for him- or herself, it is hard to work toward a solution. Long-term efforts to change come from solving a personal problem, not from following directions or adhering to recommendations. If you have ever watched "the lights come on," you know the difference.

The following example should illuminate that self-propelled action is much more powerful than adherence to directions and is integral to the model proposed here:

> By the end of high school, Eric had no idea what vocation he wanted to pursue but set off to college because he felt he was supposed to do so. Eric's interest in sports pervaded his life, from collecting cards and organizing the neighborhood to play baseball, to convincing friends to play new games he created and "broadcasting" games as he visualized them in his head. Sitting still and studying were never his forte, but he made friends easily and had a huge heart for a wide range of people. After several years of part-time college and working at a job with no future, he decided he wanted to teach physical education. This time, he had no trouble handling school, a job, and

playing ball. The change in energy and commitment to accomplish *his* goal was extraordinary to watch. Now Eric has a job that matches his unique mix of skills, interests, and personality. He teaches physical education to 5- to 13-year-olds in an inner-city school and is still organizing groups, relating to a wide range of people, making up games, staying active, *and* getting paid for it.

Many of you have probably known people who resisted suggestions from others, maybe tried some things that did not work, but bloomed when they discovered what they did want and learned how to achieve it. Successful management of obesity requires the patient's lifelong commitment to changing behavior patterns, regardless of whether medical interventions are a part of treatment. Understanding obesity, yourself, and your circumstances makes problem solving possible. Similarly, making informed decisions about care that are appropriate for each individual's unique situation requires access to information, resources, and support.

This shift in roles substantially changes the familiar format of patient-provider relationships. Historically, patients have decided what they thought about recommendations, and once they were home, they decided what they would do about them. The chronic-care model provides in-depth education to provide resources and to help equip patients for making decisions. With chronic care, it is okay to ask questions, discuss possibilities, and maybe even disagree *before* going home. Patients may not welcome the opportunity and responsibility of participating in their care, but the paradigm shift is necessary to address chronic disease. Ultimately, it is the patient's responsibility to seek answers to questions.

# The Provider's Role

In the chronic-care model, providers use their expertise to assess and explain risks, make recommendations, and offer information on treatment options and available resources. Essentially, the role of the provider shifts from one of manager to consultant. They use their extensive knowledge and experience to make recommendations but are not the decision maker. This shift in responsibility is substantial.

The model requires a different mindset, a different orientation to care than was probably provided in medical school. Because obesity is a physical symptom, physicians often feel responsible for their patients' weight reduction. Adapting to work in a chronic-care model is a paradigm shift. It requires health care providers change not just **how** they do things but **how they think** about doing things. It is important to involve physicians in both the care and change process because they are stakeholders in the transition (Hroscikoski 2006).

The chronic-care paradigm facilitates the work for everybody involved by matching the goals for both patient and provider. Medical schools have begun to teach skills in chronic-care delivery to future practitioners, supporting the necessary shift from prescribing expert to partner and preparing them to address the complex problems of chronic disease, including obesity (Stoeckle 2009).

Still, it is not surprising that even those providers who are trying to shift to a chronic-care delivery system and who are serious about helping patients integrate lifestyle changes sometimes find themselves slipping into the familiar realm of taking charge and giving directions (Anderson 2010). Many providers as well as office staff report this shift to be difficult (Carlson 1990, Lemmens 2009).

In addition to requiring that providers understand and embrace the chronic-care model, success requires collaboration and communication between everyone in the office. The shift is made easier when outcomes are measurable, job descriptions are clear, routine tasks are systematized, and appropriate training is provided (Grunbach 2004). An office that provides the team with time and space for face-to-face interactions also facilitates this change (Stroebel 2005). Learning to listen and to pose useful questions are essential skills that support the chronic-care model. Part III discusses helpful tactics for building these skills.

Effective chronic care relies on a collaborative model delivered by a health care team (Grumbach 2004). Therefore, care providers will find themselves not only collaborating with the patient in self-care goals but also with an entire team of health care professionals. It can be a daunting task, but acknowledging that every member of the team brings specific, specialized knowledge to the treatment regimen can ease this paradigm shift. The combined knowledge and skills of the entire team far surpasses the knowledge, training, experience, and skills of any single care provider.

## Table 3—Characteristics of Acute Care Versus Chronic Care

| Acute care | Chronic care |
|---|---|
| Obesity is a medical illness. The best person to treat a medical illness is a medical doctor. | Obesity is a biopsychosocial problem and a lifestyle issue. Effective treatment includes a team that offers support for lifestyle change. |
| Focuses on rapid relief of an immediate problem. | Focuses on improving function and preventing long-term complications. |
| Patient wants help to get better fast. | Patient wants help dealing with physical, emotional, and social factors contributing to an ongoing problem. |
| Possible causes are clear and relatively easy to resolve. Problem often resolves in a few weeks. | Etiology is complex, and problems can be difficult to resolve. Problem may last a lifetime. |
| Providers play an active role, whereas the patient plays a passive one. | Patients are engaged as self-managers, and the provider supports their problem-solving capabilities. |
| Patient-provider relationship is authoritarian, based on provider expertise. | Patient-provider relationship is democratic and based on shared expertise. |
| The professional is viewed as the problem solver and is responsible for diagnosis, treatment decisions, and outcome. The patient follows the professional's decisions. | The patient is viewed as the problem solver and decision maker. The professional acts as a resource and helps the patient set goals and develop a self-management plan. |

*continued on p. 48*

| Acute care | Chronic care |
|---|---|
| Appointments are short, initiated by patients to address acute problems. | Planned, regular visits are initiated by the patient. Medical interaction is part of a systematic treatment plan and involves ongoing evaluation. |
| Problems and learning needs are usually identified by professionals. | Problems and learning needs are usually identified by the patient. |
| Brief didactic education provides instructions to help patients adhere to the treatment plan. | Comprehensive self-management training provides motivation, support, and information to build patient confidence and skills for self-care. |
| The acute-care goal is behavior change. Behavioral strategies are used to increase compliance with recommended treatment. A lack of compliance is viewed as a failure of the patient and provider. | The goal of chronic care treatment is to enable patients to make informed choices. Behavioral strategies are used to help patients experiment with behavior changes of their own choosing. Behavior changes that are not adopted are viewed as experiences that can be used to develop future plans and goals. |
| Behavior change is externally motivated. | Behavior change is internally motivated. |

Adapted from Anderson (2005).

# Chapter 7

# Building the Team

To address the various factors that contribute to the obesity problem, treatment programs require the expertise of more than one professional. Given the medical, dietary, activity, and emotional factors that contribute to obesity, a physician, dietitian, exercise specialist, and psychologist can be helpful. Teams often also include a nurse who serves as a coordinator and/or an educator. A pharmacist or professional organizer may assist the team as well. Different combinations can be effective. Whether you have the opportunity to work in an onsite team to specialize in preventing and treating obesity or you practice alone and informally engage other professionals to work together, teams can offer more comprehensive obesity treatment than any individual practitioner could provide. How well the different professionals communicate and work together will affect the overall quality of treatment provided.

## What Is a Team?

A health care team is one that works together and coordinates its resources. Effective teamwork is integrated and collaborative. Effective team members see potential rather than obstacles when opinions diverge.

Health care providers have reported that it is easier to facilitate behavior change as a collaborative team than as an independent practitioner. This is especially true when working within an acute-care setting. Without the reinforcement and support of a team, it is easy to slip back into the acute-care style of relating to patients, especially when under stress.

Table 4 offers an example of a team organized to address obesity. Note that each specialty offers a unique expertise that is beyond the scope of practice for other members of the team. Whether on site or off, it is helpful to have access to a physician, dietitian, exercise specialist, and counselor. These specialists have professional training to evaluate, diagnose, and provide personalized treatment or information in key areas of weight management. However, there are several roles that anyone on the team may serve. For long-term follow-up, team members with a variety of backgrounds may serve as educators, facilitators, coordinators, or coaches. A peer counselor or coach from the community may become part of the team to discuss progress, help update short-term goals, and generally offer support between visits with the medical staff and/or psychologist.

## Table 4—Examples of Team Member Roles

| Health care professional | Best topics for referral | Area of specialization for this person* |
|---|---|---|
| Physician or primary care provider | Assess and monitor physical status and health risks. Order labs. Refer for comorbid conditions. | Diagnose disease or recommend treatments. |
| Dietitian | Assess eating patterns as they relate to comorbidities and obesity. Provide information, and help solve food-related problems. | Make specific recommendations for nutritional needs. |
| Counselor | Assess emotional and mental health and provide counseling as needed to reduce barriers to change. | Probe causes of behavior and diagnose and/or treat mental illness. |
| Exercise specialist | Assess physical flexibility, strength, and endurance. Guide activities to match patient limitations, goals, and interests. | Develop an exercise plan for people within physician-noted exercise limitations (e.g., cardiac problems, arthritis, back pain). |

*Note that these roles may be legally limited to these specialists.

| Health care professional | Best topics for referral | Area of specialization for this person |
|---|---|---|
| Educator (lifestyle-change facilitator) | | Help patients identify problems, express feelings, set realistic goals, and develop and monitor plans for change. |
| Clinical coordinator | | Coordinate care. Monitor weight, blood pressure, and lab tests. Schedule appointments. |
| All team members | | • Provide basic information in all areas<br>• Listen<br>• Acknowledge emotions<br>• Assist with problem-solving process<br>• Support patient efforts<br>• Serve as educator/lifestyle-change facilitator |

Although the specifics will vary, team members in each setting will need to define their unique and overlapping roles. If a series of classes is part of the program, each team member may teach a subject or one team member may teach all topics. There may be teams with only two or three members who refer patients to outside specialists. Professional identity is less important than having team members work with a common method and a common model for behavior change. Anderson and Funnell (2010) have found that this approach to chronic care is possible in multiple settings.

# Building a Team

Creating a collaborative team requires intentional recruiting of and training for people who are open and willing to adapt to the chronic-care paradigm. To identify possible team members, search professional directories to identify people with the credentials you need. If your focus is on diabetes, look for local members of the American Diabetes Association and/or the American Association of Diabetes Educators. To find a dietitian with a description of his or her expertise in weight management, search the Academy of Nutrition and Dietetics (www.eatright.org). To find counselors in your area with a description of their specialties, go to http://therapists.psychologytoday. com/rms/prof_search.php. Talk with colleagues and interview possible candidates. You are looking for colleagues who agree with the approach and who appear able to relate well with other team members.

To encourage collaboration and comfort with the chronic-care model, consider addressing the following issues as you build a team.

1. *Chronic Care vs. Acute Care.* The differences between chronic and acute care and the rationale for using the chronic-care model to address health problems that require behavior change were discussed in chapter 6. To what extent do potential team members understand the differences between collaborative and acute care and support the tenets of collaborative care?

2. *Consistent Work Strategy.* Is the team developing a work plan that is consistent in content and approach? Are individual team members encouraged to use their individual talents? What areas would require consistency to support a collaborative team? Here are some issues to consider while constructing the team.
    • policies and structures
    • forms
    • basic information
    • behavior change model
    • definition of obesity

3. *Required Skill Sets.* Do team members have the opportunity to learn, review, and practice the different skills needed for effective patient-

provider interactions within a chronic-care model? Proficiency in the following will be helpful in aiding patients and will help bolster the success of treatment.

- strong listening skills
- the ability to ask open-ended questions
- the willingness to be inquisitive

4. *Perception of Obesity*. What opportunities have team members had to examine their personal beliefs about obesity?

Chapter 5 discussed the rationale for treating obesity within the chronic-care paradigm. If team members are all committed to working within that paradigm, the team will have the capacity to communicate and collaborate more fully than if a member makes decisions based on the acute-care model. This paradigm shapes all decisions, big and small.

Consistency within the team simplifies the operations of the staff, but consistency in philosophy as well as in the process of patient care limits patient confusion. An excellent starting point is for the team to collaboratively determine their working definition of obesity.

# Defining Obesity

Not long ago, it was unusual to find BMI recorded in a medical chart. Even in letters of referral for weight reduction, physicians descriptively referred to patients as obese, but with no objective measurement, such as BMI or waist circumference, to indicate the degree of obesity. As stated in chapter 2, obesity is defined as abnormal and excessive fat accumulation that may impair health (WHO 2009). Different diagnostic criteria have been proposed to objectively describe obesity. BMI (a ratio of weight to height), waist circumference, and waist-to-hip ratio are currently the most common measures of obesity.

Both BMI and a measure of fat distribution (either waist circumference or waist-to-hip ratio) help calculate the risk of obesity comorbidities. To ensure consistency, the members of a collaborative team should decide which measures of obesity they will use and clearly indicate that to all members of the team.

Table 5 provides classification categories of weight based on BMI measures. The areas highlighted in light gray are the general categories most often used. This text includes the additional breakdown of the international classification for two reasons. The first is that the risk factors associated with obesity are associated with different BMI levels within some ethnic groups. The subcategories allow meaningful study within these groups while maintaining an international comparison. Secondly, as the association between BMI and risk is refined with additional data, additional cutoff points may help define treatment protocols (e.g., for drug use or bariatric surgery).

**Table 5—The International Classification of Adult Underweight, Overweight, and Obesity According to BMI**

| Classification | BMI (kg/m$^2$) | |
| --- | --- | --- |
| | Principal Cutoff Points | Additional Cutoff Points |
| Underweight | <18.50 | <18.50 |
| Severe thinness | <16.00 | <16.00 |
| Moderate thinness | 16.00–16.99 | 16.00–16.99 |
| Mild thinness | 17.00–18.49 | 17.00–18.49 |
| Normal range | 18.50–24.99 | 18.50–22.99 |
| | | 23.00–24.99 |
| Overweight | ≥25.00 | ≥25.00 |
| Pre-obese | 25.00–29.99 | 25.00–27.49 |
| | | 27.50–29.99 |
| Obese | ≥30.00 | ≥30.00 |
| Obese class I | 30.00–34.99 | 30.00–32.49 |
| | | 32.50–34.99 |
| Obese class II | 35.00–39.99 | 35.00–37.49 |
| | | 37.50–39.99 |
| Obese class III (morbid) | ≥40.00 | ≥40.00 |

From WHO (2011). In some Asian and Pacific populations, the risks associated with increasing obesity begin at a lower BMI of 22 kg/m$^2$ (WHO 2011).

# BMI

BMI is a useful tool: values are easy to calculate from commonly obtained measures of height and weight and are the same for both sexes and for adults over 20 years of age. In general, the risks associated with increasing BMI are continuous, graded, and begin at a BMI 25 kg/m², but the interpretation of BMI grading in relationship to risk may differ for different populations.

BMI does not account for the proportion of fat versus lean body mass or the location of excess fat. Athletes with increased muscle mass may have a BMI ≥30 kg/m² but little fat. In a study of college athletes, football lineman reached BMI 34 kg/m² without carrying excess fat (Ode 2007). In older people, who tend to lose muscle mass, someone may have a BMI <25 kg/m² but still carry excess adipose tissue, especially in the abdominal region. It is also true that studies have found a lower mortality risk among older adults in the overweight category than those who were normal weight or obese (Flicker 2010). These variables support caution before recommending weight loss for a 70-year-old man with a BMI of 28 kg/m². Additional measures can help provide a more complete picture.

## Waist Circumference

Because abdominal fat is strongly associated with type 2 diabetes and other metabolic risks, measuring waist circumference provides another way to assess obesity. WHO and others report evidence that waist circumference alone may provide a more practical correlate of abdominal fat distribution and the associated health risks than BMI. Waist circumference is measured at the midpoint between the lower border of the rib cage and iliac crest. A waist circumference >35 inches (>88 cm) for women and >40 inches (>102 cm) for men is a marker for obesity (Seidell 2010). As noted in chapter 2, an appropriate marker for Asian people would be lower: ≥31.5 inches (≥80 cm) for women and ≥35.5 inches (≥90 cm) for men (IDF 2006).

## Waist-to-Hip Ratio

The third measure of obesity is the waist-to-hip ratio. WHO states that a high waist-to-hip ratio has become an accepted indicator of abdominal fat accumulation. To obtain this ratio, measure the waist circumference and divide by the hip circumference. A waist-to-hip ratio >0.85 for women and >1.0 for men is a marker of obesity. In 2008, Geneva hosted an Expert Consultation on waist circumference and waist-to-hip ratio (WHO 2008). Ongoing investigations address whether BMI, waist-to-hip ratio, or waist circumference best assess obesity-related risks (Seidell 2010).

## Other Measurements

An additional measurement holds promise as a risk assessment tool. The sagittal abdominal diameter (SAD) measures the height of the abdomen while the patient is reclining on an exam table. In a small study of older men (Risérus 2004), SAD highly correlates with visceral fat and is more highly predictive of insulin resistance than any other anthropometric measurement. Larger studies found similar results with women and men (Risérus 2010). SAD is noninvasive, quick, and inexpensive but requires further testing in younger and more diverse populations to evaluate widespread reliability. To date, a SAD height >20 cm (7.9 or 8 inches) for women and >22 cm (8.7 or 9 inches) for men suggests obesity and increased metabolic risk.

Body fat is more accurately assessed by underwater weighing, not a convenient or pleasant method and certainly not practical for studying large populations. A variety of other measures offer varying degrees of accuracy, which when available, may add valuable information in clinical settings.

The point is that, despite the specificity of the calculation, BMI is an imprecise tool best used in conjunction with other measures of health risk to clinically assess and appropriately recommend treatment for individuals. To ensure consistency, members of a collaborative team should decide which measures of obesity they will use and clearly communicate decisions among all members of the team.

# Examine Personal Beliefs about Obesity

Because prejudice and stigmatization surround obesity, it is helpful for team members to reflect on and discuss their personal perspectives on these issues (Puhl 2009). It is difficult to find anyone whose perspective is not colored in some way by his or her own experiences and value systems. Discussing personal perspectives is a way to uncover subtle prejudices (Brownell 2003). Bringing them to light reduces their potential to influence future interactions.

---

### Possible Questions for Team Members to Consider

- Why are people obese? Why does a person become obese?
- Do I treat obese people differently than I treat normal-weight people?
- How do I react when I meet a severely obese person on the street?
- Do I have personal memories of being obese?
- If the team member is overweight or obese: What will it be like (or what do I think it will be like) to work professionally with people who are trying to lose weight?
- Do all obese people feel the same way about their obesity?
- Do I consider an obese person and a normal-weight person to be different in any way other than their weight?
- Do I consider obesity to be a lifestyle issue, a risk factor, or an illness?
- What is my reaction to seeing an obese person enjoying a double-dip ice cream cone or ordering super-sized fast-food meals?
- Do I have any prejudices against obese people?

---

# Teamwork Means Referrals

Collaboration with the patient is an integral part of the chronic-care model. The model also implies collaboration with other team members who share the responsibilities of patient care. Referrals to team members, whether formal or informal, keep the team functioning. Due to the multiple factors that can influence obesity, it makes sense for a new patient to meet individually with each member of the team for a comprehensive assessment. (You will find suggested issues to assess at the first and second visits in chapter 9.) Depending on the makeup of the team and the design of the program, patients may primarily relate to one member of the team as their primary facilitator.

Ideally, the program design will include routine reassessments with each team member, but any member of the team, including the patient, may request an appointment with another team member to address specific concerns. These concerns may spring from any issue that deals with the patient's health. For example, the patient may want additional information on meal planning, be experiencing abdominal pain, be bored with walking, or want to talk about family tensions. Specific team members can be called upon to provide their specialized knowledge or expertise. Referring within the team is part of being a team. This process becomes easier when team members recognize and value the unique contributions of others.

If the onsite team does not include a dietitian, exercise specialist, or psychologist, arrange for someone outside of the onsite team to be available for patient referrals. For individual practitioners, all other members of the team may be off site. In such an arrangement, communication and shared vision can be more difficult, but an outside referral is better than the patient not receiving necessary treatment. Communication may be via phone, e-mail, or fax. Efforts to provide consistent messages and make the expertise of different professionals available to patients still apply to communication that takes place outside of the clinic. Just about all of the same principles apply in such communications.

## Key Messages for Collaboration

- Assume that collaborating with professionals will improve your patients' chances of success.
- Discuss with and/or provide written information to potential referrals that describe your interest in and understanding of the chronic-care paradigm.
- Look for team members who are open to the chronic-care model and willing to communicate.
- Express your appreciation for the contributions of others.

# Nourish the Team

Working with a team can be very rewarding as well as very draining. Formal or informal, regular communications will help the team function more smoothly. Meetings may be a short briefing every morning or a longer discussion once a week. Discussions may concern issues on administration, policy, or patients. Conference calls are a way for offsite team members to participate. Expanding internet and phone technology have increased the ease and reduced the expense of communicating with others. Programs like Skype and iChat make affordable face-to-face video interactions accessible wherever there is internet access and a webcam. Whatever the topic, agendas provided before the meeting let the team know what to expect and invite preparation. Notes should be taken during the meeting and then shared, giving members a chance to make corrections and to document decisions the team has agreed upon. This "collective memory" supports follow-up.

More than 60 years later, the recommendations from Lewin (1947) to set aside time to nourish the team, evaluate the work, and get new ideas on how to work with behavior change remain valid. Hiring a consultant may help facilitate effective interactions and communication among team members (Zwarenstein 2009). Going away for a course or conference provides coworkers opportunities to reflect on their work and consider new ideas without the usual distractions. Even a group of informally coordinated professionals could meet for lunch to encourage reflection by posing the following questions.

---

### Self-Evaluation Questions for the Team

- "What have we learned during the last six months?"
- "What are we satisfied with?"
- "Is there anything about our strategy that we could improve?"
- "What are some of our successes? Why?"
- "Similarly, where did we not succeed? Why?"
- "What is the strongest contribution each team member has brought to the team in the past six months?"

---

# Insurance

The question of whether insurance will cover treatment for obesity is a persistent and pertinent one. As with any given medical problem, the extent to which insurance covers treatment can determine whether someone pursues that treatment.

Lack of health insurance, which is more prevalent among the poor, has been associated with a decline in health status (Baker 2001). Obesity is also more prevalent among the poor and is associated with a greater use and cost of medical care (Fontaine 2000). If a problem becomes acute, someone eventually absorbs those costs not directly covered by insurance. In the end, with indirect costs included, medical complications associated with obesity in the U.S. add up to more than $100 billion per year (NAASO 2006).

The North American Association for the Study of Obesity (NAASO) advocates for a medical team and health care coverage as essential for progress toward weight-management success. In its position paper, NAASO states, "even modest weight loss goals are not achievable if appropriate therapies, which include, but are not limited to, physician supervision, diet counseling, physical activity education, behavior modification, and pharmacotherapy, are not affordable. Lack of health care coverage for obesity limits treatment options, makes it difficult to obtain appropriate medical care, and drives people toward inappropriate treatment choices" (NAASO 2006).

Much money is spent on weight-loss efforts and on food, but not necessarily for effective treatments or health-building menus. People in the U.S. continue to spend about 50% of their food dollars eating out (National Restaurant Association 2010), where the food available is higher in salt, sugar, fat, calories, and cost than food prepared at home. In 2004, Americans spent $20.3 billion just on herbal and dietary supplements, which require no proof of efficacy or safety (Business Week Online 2006).

Commercial weight-loss programs and products have flooded the market with unproven promises. Programs vary greatly in the type of diet offered, duration, products used, safety, documented success, and support provided. Most are expensive and have a high attrition rate. But might some prove a helpful resource?

In a clinical trial, Rock (2010) found that when everything was free, participants lost significantly more weight using a commercial weight-loss program than the control group. Participants lost 10% of their initial weight during the first year and maintained a 7% loss at the end of year 2 using prepackaged meals and adding 150 minutes per week of exercise. The study paid for the food (worth about $5,000 retail), paid participants to attend clinic visits, and provided one-on-one counseling for 2 years. Does this suggest people will change if they are paid rather than if they have to pay for help to do so?

Many people around the world live with no health insurance. In the U.S., those with insurance receive widely inconsistent obesity-related care from their providers. The 2004 change in Medicare language first recognized obesity as a disease, making insurance coverage a possibility.

Analysis of Medicaid and state insurance laws found that although "practice guidelines recommend that clinicians screen all adult patients for obesity and offer intensive counseling and behavioral intervention to promote sustained weight loss for obese adults, the expansion of services since 2004 has been primarily bariatric surgery for the morbidly obese." State law varies dramatically from state to state, influencing the availability, services covered, and cost of obesity treatments. In 2010, surgery for obesity was covered (to some extent) in 45 states, while 20 states specifically excluded coverage for nutritional services (Lee 2010).

Bariatric surgery is expensive and not without its risks and side effects, but the limited long-term data available show a reduction in obesity-related disease and mortality after 5 years (Al Harakeh 2010). Because diet and exercise are routinely promoted as essential to successful surgical outcomes, extensive follow-up programs accompany recognized bariatric programs. It appears that surgery offers a ticket to long-term supportive care for lifestyle change that is not otherwise available.

The health care system continues to struggle as it seeks effective and economical ways to use more resources to prevent rather than treat disease. If insurance coverage does become more available, perhaps this will help people view excess weight as a medical problem and lead them to seek medical treatment before experimenting with untested commercial products.

In the meantime, here are some thoughts to consider for getting the most from available resources.

## Get the Most from Available Insurance

*Send a Bill*
For patients who have health insurance, send the bill to the insurance company regardless of whether an operator on a toll-free customer service line says it is covered or not. They are too often incorrect. Until the paperwork comes back, no one will know for sure what the coverage is. Case managers, if employed to oversee a policy, may be more able to explain the coverage and let you know the criteria and coding necessary for reimbursement.

*Use Appropriate Billing Codes*
Use appropriate and specific billing codes. Insurance may not cover

"overweight and obesity" but reimburse for "overweight," "morbid obesity," "localized adiposity," or "polyphagia." Determine whether appropriate codes are already included on your office super bill and write them in if necessary. Obviously, coding for comorbid conditions allows for higher-level billing and better reimbursement.

For individuals with diabetes, dietitians may provide and bill for two similar but distinct services.

Medical nutrition therapy (MNT) provides individual assessment, nutritional diagnosis, counseling, and follow-up using professional protocols for disease treatment. MNT is usually provided to individuals in a clinical setting. Three hours are allotted in the first year and two hours the second.

Diabetes self-management training (DSMT, also called diabetes self-management education or DSME) provides educational and training services for self-management of diabetes following nationally approved quality standards. DSMT is usually provided in a group setting. Nutrition is one of several topics (including blood glucose monitoring, exercise, medications, goal setting) addressed during the 10 hours of class time allotted during the first year of diagnosis and the 2 hours for the second year. Both services are evidence-based, require referral, and may be more medically effective together than using just one of the benefits (Daly 2009).

*Refer to Other Health Care Professionals*
Even if there is wonderful insurance coverage and top-notch billing, most primary care providers cannot remain solvent and take the time necessary to engage in weight-loss problem solving. It is valuable to monitor and explain risk factors but then refer to a dietitian and/or counseling professional for detailed information and problem solving. Physician referrals let the patient know the problem is important and makes a significant impact on his or her likelihood of scheduling an appointment. Obese individuals with exercise limitations due to hypertension or musculoskeletal problems may benefit from seeing a physical therapist to initiate realistic and safe exercise before heading to the gym on their own.

*Raise the Question of Value*
For those without insurance or with limited coverage or who resist any out-of-pocket expenses, consider asking,

"Financially, what would you have to give up to pay for treatment?"

Often, those who say they cannot afford treatment are actually saying that they do not value it as much as other things they enjoy. How much disposable income goes to eating out, movies, snacks, beer, cosmetics, or cigarettes? How much have they spent on supplements and commercial diet plans that are not supported by science?

*Despite Limited Resources, Remember To Do No Harm*
Sometimes, there is a temptation to summarize and simplify weight-loss recommendations to compensate for the uninsured visits a patient will not have. However, incorrect or partially correct information can confuse and complicate rather than help.

To provide value despite limited resources, include the following in your office visits:

- Monitor weight and waist circumference during each office visit and address risks sooner rather than later.
- Ask patients if they know the source of their extra calories. If they do, eating or drinking less can be a simple-to-understand (though perhaps difficult-to-achieve) step toward calorie reduction.
- Acknowledge that weight loss is complex and challenging, but achievable.
- Model self-care behavior. Overweight and out-of-shape health care professionals do not inspire patients to achieve better self-care.
- Keep the focus on health and weight maintenance.
- Let patients know that losing 5–10% of their current weight is medically helpful.
- Provide only current information supported by science.
- Suggest web-based programs such as My Pyramid or the Weight-control Information Network (WIN) included in the Resource section on page 196. Most people can access the internet at a local library if it is not available at home.
- Assume that patients are doing the best they can. (Scolding and scare tactics do not build confidence.)

# Chapter 8

# Create a Supportive Environment

**F**acilitating lifestyle change is a more far-ranging challenge than educational efforts to share meal planning ideas or ways to increase exercise. **Lasting lifestyle change only comes from within the person making the change.** Before anyone can consider changing his or her lifestyle, that person needs to feel respected and accepted as he or she is now. There are many prejudices against obese people. Records show that obese people are often discriminated against in education, employment, and health care (Puhl 2009). It is vital that we do not increase this social stigmatization (Brownell 2003). Providing a safe and secure environment is an important prerequisite for learning.

One way to express nonjudgmental acceptance and respect is to plan the space to comfortably accommodate obese clients. The attention to access, furnishings, privacy, and office procedures communicate provider attitudes and influence the participants' perceptions of how they are valued. A properly organized space can convey a sense of respect by the health care team and start to build the patient-provider relationship even before the first meeting.

## Access

Easy accessibility is a first step toward welcoming obese patients who may not be able to climb stairs or walk far. Providing clear, concise directions to the office prior to the appointment, especially if patients will have to navigate a ramp or an elevator, helps limit unnecessary detours and apprehension.

# Furnishings

The layout and furnishings of the waiting area and exam rooms may require some modifications to be comfortable for obese people. Although a normal-weight individual may find a narrow chair uncomfortable, for an obese patient, the chair is likely to make him or her feel conspicuous and possibly unsafe. Similarly, what if the rows of chairs are too close together and someone cannot walk through without bumping into every single chair? Avoiding these pitfalls in the clinical environment will help prevent discomforts and distractions that interfere with the purpose of the visit.

# Provide a Comfortable Waiting Area

Provide seating wide enough that even a severely obese patient can sit comfortably.

- Select furniture and rooms with enough space for the body and the legs.
- Use a check-in system that accommodates those who cannot stand for long periods of time.
- Include reading materials that depict obese people enjoying life. Include fashion magazines for people of larger sizes.

# An Exam Room that Meets the Needs of Obese Patients

Supply the room with measuring tapes, scales, blood pressure cuffs, and other equipment that are appropriate for the patient's size (Foster 2004). The measuring tape should be long enough, the cuffs wide enough, and the scale powerful enough to accommodate the patient's size and weight.

Use an exam table strong enough to hold your most obese patients without the risk of an accident. Expect that some patients may need assistance to get on and off the table safely. Ensure that no patient has reason to fear that the table (or any other feature of the exam room) will not support him or her. Breaking equipment would obviously embarrass the patient and diminish the quality of care.

Adjust the seats so provider and patient can look at each other at eye level. It is convenient to place seats at an angle, so each can have eye contact but do not have to continuously face each other directly.

Have a box of facial tissues within reach; doing so is an easy way to welcome feelings in the exam room. Discussions of lifestyle changes can uncover emotional issues and crying can sometimes accompany this.

# Privacy

Individual appointments are personal meetings. Even if the patient is dressed, he or she has a right to expect privacy. Use a system to indicate that an exam room is in use, be it a red lamp outside the door or a simple sign. There are stories from health care centers where colleagues walk in and out of the room, sometimes even without knocking, during consultations. This is inexcusable. It demonstrates an unprofessional approach to patient interaction, shows no respect for the patient's personal privacy, and shows no respect for the care provider's sessions.

# Organization

A well-organized office with trained personnel influences a patient's perception of the quality of the programs offered and his or her level of trust in the providers. Here are some issues to address when developing a strategy for the office.

- Office personnel who understand the workplace's environment and relate to the public in a courteous and professional manner do much to set the tone of the entire clinical environment.
- Consistent procedures that are tailored for the program or clinic will reduce the amount of time spent on less critical details, such as

paperwork, and reserve more time and energy for direct interaction with the patient.

- By agreeing to use shared protocols, health care providers simplify decision making, support a standard quality of care, and decrease the risk of unnecessary misunderstandings.

Though not meant to be comprehensive, these are some of the issues that help offer patients the secure environment they need in order to experiment with new behaviors and to reflect on how changes might fit into daily life. In addition to their professional expertise, the health care providers themselves influence the comfort of the patients and contribute to a secure environment. As with all patients, obese patients benefit from care providers who are mature and knowledgeable enough to offer information and recommendations without inadvertently imposing their own values and biases on the patient.

# Chapter 9

# Structuring the Care Process

*T*he manner in which we offer care may influence patient outcomes more than the care itself. The goal of this chapter is to highlight elements of the care process that communicate the character of the problem-solving model for the treatment of obesity.

## Preparation

The person scheduling appointments and the pre-visit forms is often the patient's first exposure to the practice. The format and content of the documentation forms make a first impression on the patient and influence the nature of the visit. Ideally, forms are developed, or at least selected, by those who will use them and reflect the goals of the program.

Electronic records, where available, use sophisticated software to organize patient information so that all team members can easily find reports from other team members. When all team members use the same format for documenting patient visits, the process becomes more efficient. Well-documented visits facilitate preparation for follow-up appointments and ensure that all team members can access up-to-date information on the care of the individual patient.

As mentioned in chapter 8, office equipment that fits the patient population can help patients feel more comfortable. Patients may be more tolerant of being weighed and measured if they see that the scale can clearly support them and that the tape measure will easily fit around them. Even those patients who initially refuse may eventually change their minds after learning more about the program and how the results of various measurements may help them plan and measure progress.

# The Initial Visits

One way to support the problem-solving model for behavior change is to plan two visits for the initial patient assessment. The first visit involves collecting information only and includes lab work, a behavioral assessment, and a comprehensive medical examination. The second presents and explains the results of the assessment and the treatment options available. Results of a cardiovascular risk assessment give more meaning to the numerical results of a lipid panel. Behavioral assessments help identify habits that do and do not support patient goals. The patient can use this information when deciding what changes are worth making.

## The First Visit

Greet the patient as a person, not as an obese person, with some general pleasantries. Describe your practice's philosophy of care and the goal of working with him or her as a partner in his or her care. Explain that today you will start to explore and identify the problem. You (the provider) will be listening and learning as much as you can to better understand his or her unique situation.

Funnell (2004) suggests finding out the patient's reason for being there by asking open-ended questions like:

- What prompted you to come see us?
- What are your hopes for this visit?
- What would you like to see happen in the next few weeks or months?
- What do you most need from us to help you make that happen?

The first visit for the treatment of obesity naturally includes baseline measurements of obesity. These measurements can trigger emotional landmines. More than one person has refused to seek medical care because they did not want to be weighed. For obese patients, stepping on a scale and answering questions about their weight can be especially difficult. Many have had painful experiences associated with body weight, body shape, and eating habits. Some are ashamed of their weight and view their size as a personal failure that they are not eager to validate. For some patients, it takes great courage to step on the scale, and others simply refuse to do it. Respecting the patient's feelings will help patients build confidence in lifestyle change more than coercing compliance. Gently approach the task of measuring obese people.

A patient who has not stepped on the scale for years may be willing to do so with some support. Some counselors have reported that it helps to hold hands with the patient just before he or she steps on the scale and then sometimes staying with the patient while he or she cries after learning the result. It is just as important that care providers address the patients' *response* to learning about their risk factors as it is for patients to learn about risk factors. Although requesting measurements may cause discomfort, it may also encourage patients to face the problems that negatively affect their health. Some people will be relieved to get their concerns out in the open. Until someone can face and accept his or her current circumstances, no matter how painful these might be, he or she is ill prepared to plan for the future. Becoming aware and expressing emotions is a positive step toward making lifestyle changes.

The box on page 72 suggests information to gather in an initial assessment. One of the difficulties of treating people with chronic obesity is the complexity of the many issues that may contribute to the problem. A comprehensive assessment helps detect problem areas and focus discussion. Obtaining a medical history and a physical require a physician or other primary care provider, but collecting the other information may be delegated to other members of the team.

## The First Visit: Gathering Information

Topics that are standard or typically included in a comprehensive physical:

**Medical history:** diagnosis, treatment, and status
Physical assessment:
- Laboratory tests
- Physical measurements: blood pressure, height, weight, and waist circumference
- Current medications and treatments
- Other medications, e.g., dietary supplements, alternative/complementary medicines
- Other health care providers

**Social history:** psychosocial factors, family life, work life

Additional key topics in addressing obesity:
- Weight history
  - Onset of excess weight
  - Former weight-reduction activities and their outcomes
  - Perception of the cause and of the impact excess weight has on daily life
- Dietary habits
  - Timing of meals and/or snacks
  - Frequency of dining out and eating convenience food
  - Amount of caloric liquids consumed
- Physical activity
  - Type, frequency, time, and intensity of current activities
  - Longevity and enjoyment of activity
  - Limitations

Having patients complete assessment forms before the visit can help providers quickly access key information and identify areas for follow-up

STRUCTURING THE CARE PROCESS

questions. Behavior-type questions may be integrated into the general medical assessment form or appear in a standalone questionnaire. To encourage completion, design patient assessment forms that are easy to finish by using multiple choice, rating scales, or other short answer questions.

Most of the key obesity topics on the previous page could be included in a questionnaire. Hopefully these weight history questions can help you and your patient uncover important lessons from any previous experiences with weight gain and loss.

- Who is concerned about your weight (you, family member, friend, doctor, other)?
- Do you want to lose weight now? How much?
- How old were you when you or someone else first became concerned about your weight?
- During what periods of your life were you gaining weight?
- Have you tried to lose weight?
- If yes, what have you tried? (may use multiple choice, including other) (Follow-up verbal questions might be: what worked, what did not, what did you learn? What support did you have for losing weight?)
- How many times have you lost weight and then regained it (0–3, 4–5, 6–10, more than 10 times)?

Topics addressing cause, impact, and motivation are topics for discussion. Use these discussions to try to help patients identify the benefits of weight loss (i.e., changing their lifestyle) that would make doing so worth the effort. Look for assessment-type questions to stimulate dialog in subsequent chapters. Examples of assessment forms are in the Appendix: Meal Habits, Eating Schedule Timeline, Risky Situations, and Reasons for Overeating. An extensive eating habits inventory is available at http://www. balancedweightmanagement.com/Your Eating Habits Inventory.htm.

# The Second Visit

After the first and before the second appointment, the team compiles the information collected during the first visit to share with the patient during the second visit. Use of a standardized form to compare patient results with published norms and recommended ranges helps keep the report objective. If the team chooses to, use of a risk assessment tool to evaluate risks from a combination of data may further help patients understand the implications of their results, but this adds further expense to collecting and processing the information. To complete the record for patient feedback, note whether the patient's current medications may be contributing to weight gain and summarize significant findings from weight, diet, and physical activity history.

---

### The Second Visit:
### Assessment Results and Treatment Options

The first part of this visit requires sharing the results of objective tests.
- Compare physical data with normal levels.
  - ◆ Lab tests
  - ◆ BMI
  - ◆ Blood pressure
  - ◆ Waist circumference
- Review risk-assessment profile.
- If current medications are known to contribute to weight gain, explain this and see if other options are available.

The second part requires summarizing the subjective information collected on these three topics and confirm its accuracy.
- Weight history
- Dietary habits
- Physical activity

---

The first part of the second visit involves sharing the results from objective tests administered during the first meeting. It is important to keep this delivery factual and avoid possible judgmental language, such as "good" and "bad," which can communicate a value assessment. The second part of this visit requires the care provider to summarize any information that has not or cannot be validated by tests or evaluations and confirm accuracy.

Results from the assessment and the patient's response to the assessment provide fuel for planning change. Depending on a patient's risk factors, open-ended questioning can help clarify understanding and stimulate ideas for the next steps in beginning lifestyle change.

---

### Possible Brainstorming Questions for Behavioral Therapy

- Did you learn anything from the results of your assessment that you did not already know?
- Do you have questions about the results or what they mean?
- How do you feel about the assessment results?
- What concerns you the most?
- Is there anything you want to change? If so, what? What would need to happen to make that change?
- Would you like help? I can refer you to someone (a team member) who can give you more information and support for implementing that change.

---

# Deciding to Change

The decision to take action is in sole possession of the patient. Typically, responses fall into one of three categories in regard to behavior change. One response is that the patient is happy to participate. Other patients are uncertain whether they want to take the steps in changing their lifestyles. Some patients do not want to participate at all. Follow-up for members of the first group is clear; refer them to an appropriate team member for further consultation.

There can be many reasons why a patient hesitates to attempt change. Avoidance is one common reason. Previous attempts at behavior change can shape expectations, as can instances wherein behavior change was forced upon the patient. As one of my patients recently told me, "As long as I don't know my weight, I don't have to address the issue. As soon as I know it, I have to decide on a behavior change that I don't know if I will be able to fulfill in the long run."

The possibility of failure, or the remembrance of failure, often encourages patients to avoid therapy. In situations such as this, it is often best to remind the patient that behavior change is a process and that it takes a long time. Emphasize that change will not come instantly and that occasional missteps (which do not mean failure) are acceptable and more or less expected. In this case, the care provider can accentuate the role of realistic goals and small steps in ensuring long-lasting behavior change. Hesitant patients may benefit from a referral to someone else in the team, if needed, to receive current information about specific lifestyle and behavior change possibilities. Some will be relieved to learn that life-style changes need not be drastic and that they can choose what changes suit their present situation and needs.

Respect the decision of people who are not interested in committing to behavior change at this time. Affirm their right to decide. Any attempt to force behavior change on a patient is more likely to discourage follow-up than encourage participation. Even unspoken expectations from providers undermine patient confidence and increase stress levels. Ultimately, pressuring behavior change on a patient is counterproductive because stress often increases food intake. If the patient rejects the idea of behavior change, say something along these lines: "I understand that you are not interested in making changes right now. If you change your mind, please know you are welcome to seek us out so we can work together on this in the future."

There are some positive aspects to this scenario. You have let the patient know that the health care team is available to help solve his or her prob-lem and that the team can be seen as a valuable resource, not a nagging group of doctors, nurses, dietitians, and so forth. Regardless of whether the patient is interested in behavior change right now, perhaps you have planted a seed. He or she has experienced the care provider respecting his or her individual decisions about self-care. Additionally, the patient has seen that honesty is appreciated and acknowledged. The patient could have easily lied and simply not followed through on the behavior change recommendations. With a strong foundation for the patient-provider rela-tionship, the patient might call several months later or voluntarily bring up the issue of lifestyle change during the next annual checkup.

One way to track the development of obesity and its associated risk factors is to establish a team policy to measure BMI and waist circumfer-ence at every appointment. If BMI or waist circumference results exceed the normal cutoff values (BMI $\geq 25$ kg/$m^2$ and waist circumference $\geq 35$ inches for women and $\geq 40$ inches for men), then the patient can be offered a follow-up appointment to assess related risk factors.

An annual reassessment of risk factors has great potential as a teach-ing tool for patients in a primary care office as well as in an obesity clinic. Information about their risks is updated and reinforced. Health care pro-fessionals can confirm and accept patient responses to elevated risk fac-tors. They can also answer questions about available support for behav-ior change efforts. Each following assessment, regardless of how the patient responds to the suggestion of behavior change, will strengthen the relationship and possibly encourage him or her to pursue lifestyle modification.

Ultimately, however, the patient is the only person who decides whether to accept help in any form. As difficult as it is for us as care pro-viders to admit that we are not in control, we do serve the patient's best interests when we accept, acknowledge, and respect the patient's right to choose.

# Part III

# Tools to Facilitate Self-Care

# Chapter 10

# Problem Solving:
# An Introduction

I n the traditional acute-care model, professionals define the patient's problem. Health professionals see excess weight as a problem because it is a medical risk. In a collaborative problem-solving model, the patient defines the problem and may view the excess weight quite differently than does the health professional.

Traditional weight-reduction programs focus their efforts on the weight-reduction period and the number of pounds lost. Many programs, designed by both commercial and health care organizations, provide a structure for weight-loss plans, information about food, and meal planning support. Some offer prepared foods to simplify planning. Most people who follow the plans as directed lose weight, but eventually they become unwilling or unable to continue following the meal plan. Even though they may continue to apply some of the information they have learned, they regain some or all of the lost weight. They learned a system but did not learn to solve the problem.

To support sustained weight control, an alternative approach is to focus efforts toward changing behaviors that contribute to weight gain rather than on the weight itself. It is possible to lose weight in a variety of ways that do not improve health, such as skipping meals or omitting required nutrients. Weight may fluctuate over the short term due to factors beyond an individual's control, such as constipation or a change in medication. For most patients (and most individuals, too), everyday issues present the major obstacles to making lasting behavior change. Helpful problem-solving skills offer a way to overcome obstacles.

Sometimes, patients find that their significant others pressure them about the number of pounds lost during their weight-loss program. This social pressure does not contribute to healthy attitudes toward the lengthy process of losing weight, and patients may need help to respond constructively. You can help them formulate responses to situations like these. For example, you can suggest that the patient say something like: "For me, my efforts are more about improving my habits than about losing weight. I am learning about why I eat too much. I am changing some old habits that helped me become this size. So, I am trying to change my lifestyle. I already feel better and trust that the weight I do lose will last."

For patients, changing behavior requires a skill set different from that required for following a care provider's usual instructions, such as taking a prescription medication. Remembering to take medication as directed requires some adjustment but is minor compared to the number of changes required to improve eating habits. Usual eating habits develop over a lifetime and are reinforced by current circumstances. Changing behavior means identifying the specific cues that prompt and the barriers that discourage an individual's positive behavior change.

In a collaborative model that emphasizes strong problem-solving skills, the patient is allowed to test his or her hypotheses and, through experience, learn what works and what does not. Learning and developing new eating habits is a gigantic undertaking. It is not a simple task in which a person learns new techniques to be used at restaurants and holiday parties; it affects our whole lifestyle and all social interactions. As care providers, we hope not to (or guard against) inadvertently suggest(ing) that assimilating new behaviors will be easy. For example, if we recommend that a patient simply select healthier options off a restaurant menu and we present it as if it is a simple task, how well will the patient succeed at behavior change? What if that person normally enjoys a decadent dessert with his or her grandchild and has been doing this for years—so long that it has become family tradition? The wide-ranging consequences of these behavior changes must be acknowledged and examined by both the patient and the health care team.

The skills, training, and education provided to patients in order to accomplish behavior change have to match their needs. To be effective, this essential "behavior change toolbox" builds on the patient's current knowledge, skills, and abilities. The toolbox must also be integrated with the patient's current frame of reference. If an individual does not know how to read a food label, then we should not instantly teach them how to develop meal plans based on point systems. Likewise, instituting an exercise routine is important, but if the patient has not rigorously exercised in a few years, it is more helpful to give them a pedometer and request that they start using a walking log than it is to sign them up at the gym. Our goal is to provide a behavior change toolbox with all of the necessary tools a patient will need to meet realistic goals, including ones that are useful for handling social situations.

Instituting behavior change requires planning and preparation. It asks an individual to reflect on which behaviors to change in order to help him or her best achieve goals without decreasing mental, physical, or psychosocial well-being. If an individual satisfies his personal needs for comfort with food, he may have to learn new ways to satisfy those needs. If relationships with family, friends, or colleagues are sustained and nourished through shared meals, a person's decision to eat differently will affect those relationships. Changes such as these will require the patient to learn new ways of interacting with significant others. This, of course, is no easy task.

# The Professional's Role

The responsibility of deciding what changes to make and for carrying out those changes remains with the patient. The health professional's responsibility is to support the patient's problem-solving abilities and thus help him or her overcome the practical problems that could threaten lasting change. Patients and professionals are equally responsible in this process, but for different issues. The professional's capacity lies in improving our patients' problem-solving skills. Mastering a practical model for solving problems increases self-efficacy and motivation for further participation in health-related behavior change efforts (Battersby 2010).

Professionals support their patients' problem-solving skills by providing a secure environment, maintaining expertise in areas of specialization, and asking appropriate questions. A secure environment is one where the patient can reflect on his or her situation and feel free to consider different possible solutions to a problem without external pressure. It is one in which the patient can feel free of judgment and discrimination regardless of his or her size or personal lifestyle choices. To offer a secure, emotionally safe learning environment requires that health professionals maintain a neutral response to patient decisions and resist the temptation to provide unsolicited advice. This may be the most difficult task for health professionals. To remain neutral requires refraining from offering praise or criticism, so patients have the opportunity to discover what they actually think, feel, and want to do.

Health care professionals require no less training or skill to work in a chronic-care setting where patients identify and solve problems than in a more traditional setting where providers diagnose and treat. Professional expertise is just as necessary to support and teach others in problem solving as it is in an independent setting. Information is essential to problem solving, but in the chronic-care model, it is provided in response to patients' questions and concerns as they arise rather than on the professional's timetable. Various members of the health care team can usually answer general questions, but they can also refer patients to another team member when a particular specialty is required to respond with the accuracy and detail requested. If team members cannot provide the information requested, it is their responsibility to help the patient find that information elsewhere.

A key responsibility for professionals working in a chronic-care setting is to ask questions that help patients find their own answers. Appropriate questions can stimulate patients' insight into their own behaviors, feelings, attitudes, needs, and beliefs. Stimulating such insight is necessary for successful problem solving and for making sustainable behavior changes. For many clinicians, asking open-ended questions and having to hear about feelings may be a difficult or uncomfortable situation. In such instances, it will help the entire health care team if they seek further training or guidance to use strategies and tactics for motivational interviewing and questioning.

There are at least three reasons for developing this skill. First, not addressing the emotional underpinnings of a behavior interferes with the possible success of behavior change. Second, emotions are the fuel for action. As people become aware of uncomfortable feelings or emotions related to their current behavior, the energy for change increases. This is an opportunity to strengthen internal motivation. Third, experiencing feelings and emotions that interfere with behavior change does not constitute mental illness or require a psychiatric referral—many of these issues can be addressed by the members of the health care team. As with issues of nutrition, exercise, and medication, there is a basic level of coaching expertise that the team can share and a more sophisticated level of expertise held by the specialist, e.g., a psychologist.

What follows is a model of ground-level ideas and questions that anyone on the team might use to support problem solving. In brief, there are five basic steps to facilitate behavior change using the problem-solving model.

1. Clearly identify the problem.
2. Explore feelings related to the problem.
3. Set realistic goals.
4. Develop a plan of action and behavior change.
5. Evaluate the plan.

# Chapter 11

# Step One:
# Identify the Problem

**B**ecoming aware of a problem is the first step toward solving it. This step improves awareness by specifically defining the problem. The second step (addressed in chapter 12) further clarifies the problem by exploring the emotions associated with the problem and with what it means to solve the problem. Increased awareness of a problem behavior strengthens the patient's power to change that behavior.

The key element in supporting patients' problem solving is to help them clearly identify the problem behaviors and determine the steps necessary to resolve them. To help the patients' awareness of a problem, our responsibility may require asking uncomfortable questions. Evading issues that appear to be sensitive for or are avoided by the patient does not help them gain understanding or change a problem behavior. If it appears that an issue may be sensitive for the patient or that the issue has long gone unaddressed, some careful questioning may be in order. In situations such as these, open-ended questioning generally proves helpful. For example, the care provider can ask, "May I ask you about something associated with your relationship life?" Remember, however, that it is the patient's right to not answer a question if he or she so desires.

The members of the health care team will best serve their patients by guarding against any attempt to break down a patient's resistance and walls of defense. These walls only fall when the patient feels secure and does not need them any longer. Members of the team can advocate change, but they cannot enact change for the patient. The health care team's role is to maintain a nonjudgmental attitude. Our job is not to judge or determine what is right or wrong, good or bad, but to support the patient's problem-solving ability. This is achieved by respecting the patient's views and by trying to understand the patient's perspective. This supportive stance is demonstrated by asking the patient questions in order to help him or her reflect on problem behaviors. Similarly, we can guide patients in their efforts to address problem behaviors, but we cannot simply mandate a treatment regimen. Ownership of the problem and its solution lead to successfully treating it, but only the patient can take control of these issues.

# The Patient Identifies the Problem

The patient's perspective defines the problem. Because the patient will be responsible for the everyday decisions and actions required to change behavior, he or she also chooses which problem is most important to address.

There are many levels and areas for defining a problem associated with obesity. Obesity-associated problems could be a metabolic risk factor, such as hypertension or impaired glucose tolerance, or a physical symptom, such as pain in the knees, back, or feet due to excess weight overloading the skeleton. The patient could also define the problem as behavioral, such as excessive eating in certain situations, which compounds the obesity problem. Problems may involve difficulties with relationships; for example, perhaps the patient's mother-in-law offers cake all the time and becomes annoyed when it is refused. Other behavioral issues may be related to

- social gatherings
- engaging in physical activity
- making appropriate food choices in the grocery store
- job performance
- obesity dominating everyday living
- eating in public places
- enjoying leisure time
- feeling confident in eating situations

## Case Study 1
### Further Exploration Uncovers Mary's Problem

Mary, 60 years old, has been trying to lose weight through meal planning, but it isn't working as well as she'd like. Therefore, she recently added a problem-solving session to determine what obstacle is interfering with her losing weight. She defines the problem as such: the regular meal habits that she has successfully introduced have not resulted in any weight reduction. She carefully and thoroughly describes her meal plan to her dietitian. Besides the meals, she has two planned snacks, just as the dietitian recommended at a previous consultation. To confirm what Mary has just said and to avoid any misunderstanding, the dietitian repeats what Mary told her. Both Mary and the dietitian consider it strange that Mary has not lost any weight. They are looking for a clue as to why Mary has not lost weight.

The dietitian asks Mary to repeat her meal plan and listens very carefully. This time, she hears Mary's expression "empty calories," which she did not catch the first time, partly due to Mary's brief attitude, lowered voice, and heightened speed when saying it. Here's what Mary actually said: "And then we have those 'empty calories,' but they don't count since they are empty." The dietitian suspected that these "empty calories" were probably the link to the missing weight loss.

If identifying the reason for the lack of weight loss still remained an issue, then the patient could keep a food record for a couple of days (see page 91). The patient writes down what, when, and how much he or she eats and the reason for eating. Keeping a food record can be beneficial because it requires that the patient pay attention to his or her food choices and increases self-knowledge, possibly unearthing the problem behavior. A food record also provides the dietitian with another tool for helping the patient.

Instructing patients to add up the calorie content of their foods provides more information and may help them understand why they are

*(continued)*

obese. An estimate of energy expenditure compared with energy intake further clarifies this picture.

# Help the Patient Define the Problem

The foundation of the problem-solving process is the successful definition of behavioral problems. The problem-solving process gives hope to the patient. The process offers patients the support they need to increase their awareness of problem behaviors and, if necessary, to act on a problem previously neglected, avoided, or denied. As the patient's perceived ability to solve problems increases, hope and the potential to solve further problems increases (Stuifbergen 1994).

Here are some general guidelines for helping the patient define his or her problem.

- Be curious and inquisitive.
- Respect and accept the patient's definition of the problem.
- If there are many problems identified, ask which one the patient considers to be the most important.
- Never underestimate what can be uncovered by asking open-ended and nonjudgmental questions.

## Questions to Help the Patient Define the Problem

- What does knowing about your risk factors make you think about?
- What concerns you most about changing your lifestyle?
- What do you see as the biggest problem in achieving lifestyle change?
- What do you find is the hardest part of changing your eating habits?
- What part of your current lifestyle is causing you the most problems?

Adapted from Anderson (2005).

Table 6—Blank Food Record/Diary

Name: _____                                        Date: _____

| Time/meal/place | Description of food and beverage, one item on each line | Amount | Calories (kcal) | Notes |
|---|---|---|---|---|
| | | | | |
| | | | | |
| | | | | |
| | | | | |
| | | | | |
| | | | | |
| | | | | |
| | | | | |
| | | | | |
| | | | | |
| | | | | |
| | | | | |
| | | | | |
| | | | | |
| | | | | |
| | | | | |
| | | | | |
| | | | | |

**Table 7—Sample Food Record**

**Name:** Melanie Brown

**Date:** Monday, 5/6

| Time/meal/place | Description of food and beverage, one item on each line | Amount | Calories (kcal) | Notes |
|---|---|---|---|---|
| 7:25 a.m. Breakfast Table in kitchen | Juice | 3/4 cup | | |
| | Bread | 3 slices | | |
| | Butter | 1 Tbsp | | |
| | Cheese, 26% fat | 3 oz. | | |
| | Coffee | 1 cup | | Too much? |
| | Milk | 1/2 cup | | |
| 11 a.m. Snack At my desk | Coke | 12-oz can | | |
| | Coffee | 1 cup | | |
| | Milk (2% fat) | 6-oz glass | | |
| 2 p.m. Lunch McDonald's | Quarter Pounder with cheese | 1 | | Hungry, late lunch |
| | French Fries | medium | | |
| | Coke | medium, 21 oz | | |
| | Apple Pie | 1 | | |
| 6:00 p.m. Going home from work In the car | Chocolate | 3 oz | | Tired |
| 8:00 p.m. Home | Bread | 5 slices | | Tired |
| | Butter | 2 Tbsp | | |
| | Cheese | 8 slices | | |
| | Ham, lean, roasted | 3 oz | | |
| | Beer, 3.5% alcohol | 2 cans | | |
| | Apple | large | | |

**Table 8—Sample Food Record with Calories Included**

Name: Melanie Brown

Date: Monday, 5/6

| Time/meal/place | Description of food and beverage, one item on each line | Amount | Calories (kcal) | Notes |
|---|---|---|---|---|
| 7:25 a.m. Breakfast Table in kitchen | Juice | 3/4 cup | 90 | |
| | Bread | 3 slices | 3 × 80 = 240 | |
| | Butter | 1 Tbsp | 100 | |
| | Cheese, 26% fat | 3 oz. | 3 × 100 = 300 | Too much? |
| | Coffee | 1 cup | 0 | |
| | Milk | 1/2 cup | 60 | |
| 11 a.m. Snack At my desk | Coke | 12-oz can | 150 | |
| | Coffee | 1 cup | 0 | |
| | Milk (2% fat) | 6-oz glass | 90 | |
| 2 p.m. Lunch McDonald's | Quarter Pounder with cheese | 1 | 530 | Hungry, late lunch |
| | French Fries | medium | 450 | |
| | Coke | medium, 21 oz | 225 | |
| | Apple Pie | 1 | 265 | |
| 6:00 p.m. Going home from work In the car | Chocolate | 3 oz | 400 | Tired |
| 8:00 p.m. Home | Bread | 5 slices | 5 × 80 = 400 | Tired |
| | Butter | 2 Tbsp | 2 × 100 = 200 | |
| | Cheese | 8 slices | 8 × 100 = 800 | |
| | Ham, lean, roasted | 3 oz | 125 | |
| | Beer, 3.5% alcohol | 2 cans | 2 × 146 = 292 | |
| | Apple | large | 130 | |

## Case Study 2

### Carol Identifies Her Problem as Stopping Water Aerobics Classes

Carol, 32 years old, initially defined her problem as her entire life. "Everything is a mess," she said. She cares for her two children and works full time. After her divorce two years ago, Carol joined Weight Watchers and lost 60 pounds. Then she regained the 60 pounds plus another 10. It is easy to understand why Carol gains weight when she describes her day.

Carol is up at 6:00 a.m., feeds the pets, wakes the children, and serves them breakfast before she goes to work. Most of Carol's coworkers are weight-conscious women who bring her articles on diets, which they urge her to follow. Carol admits that she can feel their accusing eyes watching her during lunch. During afternoon coffee, they argue with Carol when she declines a cookie, telling her that one cookie will not matter. These breaks are hardly a moment of relaxation for Carol; she feels too much pressure from her colleagues. Because she does not want to confront her colleagues' comments on her eating habits and obesity, Carol usually skips lunch and spends her lunch hour at her desk. In the afternoon, she occasionally gets some donuts and coffee from the cafeteria. Carol buys dinner on her way home. By that time, she is so hungry from skipping lunch and from frustration that she purchases a piece of chocolate or some other snack along with dinner. At home, everyone is in a hurry. The children are hungry and have to leave soon for their lessons or sports activities. Fresh vegetables take too much time to prepare, so Carol and her family eat what is convenient rather than what is nutritious. After Carol drives the children to and from their activities, it is time for their homework. Meanwhile, Carol takes care of the household chores. By 10:00 p.m., with the children in bed, it finally is "Carol time." She loads a tray with cheese and crackers, sandwiches, chips, sweets, and ice cream. Then she lies on her bed, watches TV, and finally relaxes. Carol has lost control over her eating and does not know where to start to regain command.

When asked to prioritize her problems, Carol quickly points out the moment when things seemingly spiraled out of her control. She used to attend a water aerobics class, which she had begun while attending Weight Watchers. When attending these classes, Carol felt good; she met other women in a nice environment and was glad to be doing something that improved her well-being. Unfortunately, due to her busy schedule, Carol had to stop attending these classes. Carol felt she betrayed herself by quitting the one thing that made her feel good and was good for her.

After identifying her problem behaviors and looking for ways that would help her attain her weight-reduction goals, Carol decided to start by increasing her physical activity. She found a friend in her weight-reduction group willing to take the water aerobics class with her one night a week. Carol then started to look at the food labels on what she ate, and now she does not buy food with more than 15% fat. At Carol's last visit, she was still enjoying the water aerobics class one night a week with her friend. She managed to eat more regularly, including breakfast every day. She also decided a job change would be good for her. However, with her current situation, she had neither the time nor the energy to address this, but decided to be open to possibilities. In six months, she decided that she would reconsider looking for a new job.

Unsolicited "suggestions" from coworkers increased Carol's emotional response and intensified her negative behavior. When excessive eating is due to emotional reasons, it is important that the patient alone discovers which emotions and needs precipitate eating. The care provider can guide but not mandate. Such guidance allows the patient to do the hard work and leads to a sense of discovery and acknowledgment. If he or she feels some responsibility for unearthing it, the patient will find that he or she "owns" the problem.

## Some Common Reasons
## Given by Patients for Excessive Eating

- Poor character (often undefined)
- Eating too much candy, chocolate, cookies, chips, or ice cream
- Big portions of food
- Social eating
- Late evening eating
- Eating too many sandwiches
- Feelings of depression
- Between-meal snacking
- Difficulty resisting something that tastes good
- Difficulty ordering healthy meals

- Eating provides comfort
- Feelings of fatigue and weakness
- Worry
- Anxiety
- Eating is a reward
- Financial reasons
- Smoking cessation
- Alcohol use
- Stress
- Anger
- Pain
- Boredom
- Overwhelmed

## Case Study 3
### Taking Time to Identify Feelings

Danielle, 42 years old, has participated in a weight-reduction group for six months. She has worked on her eating habits and has experienced some success. She now regularly eats both breakfast and dinner but still skips lunch. Danielle has a stressful job and often has to use her lunch break to see customers.

During one of her meetings with her group, she described an event that happened recently. After a meeting with an executive whom she wanted to impress, Danielle felt that something was not right, but at the moment, couldn't pinpoint why. As Danielle was driving to her next appointment, she felt that something was very wrong and wished she could turn back the clock and repeat the meeting. She felt a strong craving for something warm, soft, and good to replace the emptiness she felt in her stomach. She stopped the car to have a piece of chocolate and a hot dog. To be sure that the negative feelings would not affect her next meeting, she got two chocolate bars for the road.

The sensations Danielle felt were feelings of shame, disappointment, and frustration from making a bad impression (or so she thought) during the first meeting. However, she did not recognize those feelings right after the meeting and instead soothed her feelings with food. Her feelings became clearer later that evening, when she had time to reflect. Danielle realized that her horrible feelings were created by stress. Stress was what pushed her to hurry to her next appointment rather than think about the first meeting, and it was that same stress that distracted her so much that she could not connect her bad feelings from the meeting with the dark hole she felt in her stomach.

Learning from this experience, Danielle decided to schedule a short break after every meeting to unload uncomfortable experiences and reflect on difficult feelings that could induce cravings and increase the risk of excessive eating. Furthermore, this experience gave Danielle the emotional fuel she needed to include a lunch break in her daily dietary pattern. This would make it easier for her to trace her cravings and determine whether these cravings arose from hunger or some other source.

When Danielle was able to observe her problem behavior as information and without judgment, she could then use that information to help her solve the problem.

## Case Study 4
### Charlie's Unstructured Eating and High-Fat, Low-Fiber Diet

Charlie, 52 years old, is married with three children. He started to gain weight when he stopped playing soccer. He developed abdominal obesity and hypertension and eventually had cardiac bypass surgery and two

*(continued)*

heart attacks. Due to the side effects of his antihypertensive medication, Charlie developed erectile dysfunction, making his and his wife's sexual lives almost nonexistent. Charlie felt stressed most of the time. On most days, he worked overtime and still had to bring work home. He coached soccer after work three or four days a week, too. On the way from work to soccer, Charlie would often stop for fast food, usually hamburgers and fries or pizza. One of his daughters is overweight, and she and Charlie tried new diets together without success. Charlie's wife is thin, and he felt that she did not support his efforts to follow healthier eating habits. She rarely served vegetables with meals and often left a bowl of peanuts for him on the table near the TV. Charlie found it very hard to resist these snacks.

Charlie said that his stressful life was the primary barrier keeping him from having regular meals and eating healthy food. He saw no way to change the situation at work that substantially contributed to his stress levels. When his annual checkup identified impaired glucose tolerance, the doctor referred Charlie to a diabetes education program open to people with prediabetes. His wife came with him to get information on lifestyle changes in the hope of lowering his risk for diabetes. They met with a dietitian and participated in an exercise class. By working from the same information and by realizing that not everything had to be done at once, they became committed to reducing Charlie's diabetes risk. Charlie felt that his everyday stress level (i.e., his primary barrier) created his main eating problems: unstructured eating with a high-fat, low-fiber diet.

The first change Charlie made was to improve his fast-food choices. He decided that when he's going to eat a hamburger he'll skip the fries, and he'll only order pizza with one meat topping. He started wearing a pedometer to see how much he walked every day and added 2,000 steps to his initial 4,500 steps per day by pacing the sidelines during soccer practice. His wife added vegetables to their meals, which Charlie enjoyed. Later, Charlie began to pack a sandwich and an apple to eat between work and soccer practice and started sharing a large salad with his wife when he got home late. He gradually increased his steps up to 8,000 a day, worked fewer hours, and lost nearly 10 pounds.

Follow-up with the physician and with the education program helped Charlie continue with his good work and build on his efforts for another year and a half. Then his wife became ill, and his insurance would no longer pay for follow-up visits for weight loss. Charlie returned to working more hours and began gaining weight. His increase in risk factors led to a return of elevated glucose and a diagnosis of diabetes within a year. A couple of years later, his health forced him into early retirement.

Last time we met, Charlie's schedule was less busy and stressful. He told me that he did not think it was as important to keep busy anymore. "I have realized that if I want to enjoy life I have to slow down," he said. "I'm not as involved with soccer, and sometimes I am able to say 'no' instead of 'yes,' as I used to. I try to keep my evenings free, and since I am retired, I do not carry the 24-hours-a-day responsibility to my former customers as I did. Still, if things come up that no one else will do, I feel I have to take them on."

Charlie's problems with health and behavior change are hardly unique. Although he experienced many setbacks, with the proper amount of support, he was able to make and maintain positive changes, even under very stressful conditions. His health care team was supportive, patient, and nonjudgmental, allowing Charlie to change at his own pace. Moreover, his situation shows how a lack of insurance can obstruct behavior change and increase the chances that a preventable risk factor can become a chronic health problem. Charlie later told us how much the support he received meant to his behavior change efforts and how he regretted that he had stopped due to lack of insurance coverage.

## Case Study 5
### Bill's Chocolate Impulse

Bill, 53 years old, suffered a cerebral hemorrhage two years ago and is still on sick leave. He tried to return six months ago but found that working was too stressful. Bill believes his high cholesterol and blood

*(continued)*

pressure caused his brain damage and considers himself lucky to have a second chance. Bill set a goal to gradually lose weight and thus reduce his hypertension and cholesterol.

When working, Bill had been the head of his department. If he was not working, he was on his way to or from a job. He enjoyed the adrenaline kicks and now misses that part of the job. Recently, Bill learned his company was cutting expenses, and they offered him an early retirement pension. He was shocked, but after thinking it through, he accepted the offer. Bill had adjusted his lifestyle and wanted to keep stress levels at a minimum. He was still sensitive, easily stressed, and required more time to complete some tasks than before the hemorrhage. He did not want to keep his job and jeopardize his health.

Meanwhile, Bill bought a house outside the city, was planning his garden for the coming season, and had begun a relationship. Bill became careful about his food choices and paid more attention to the quality of his food. Slowly but steadily, he began to lose weight. Being very practical and knowing that maintaining a healthy weight is usually more difficult than losing weight, Bill decided to let his weight stabilize for a while after he had lost 15 pounds. Later, he could start with a new period of weight reduction.

To his surprise, Bill began to gain a little weight during that maintenance period. The culprit was chocolate. For some reason, there were certain occasions when he simply could not resist buying chocolate. He associated the craving with times when he felt that certain people disappointed him or made him angry. In these situations, chocolate provided comfort. Then Bill recalled how he used to have chocolate bars on his way home from work. After recognizing this pattern and addressing it, the "chocolate thing" stopped. Bill continues to maintain his weight and plans to start a new weight-reduction period in two months.

As illustrated by these case studies, although obesity is a widespread problem, keys to improvement are as unique as the individual facing it.

# Chapter 12

# Step Two: Explore Feelings

*A*fter identifying the problem, the next step is to explore and address the feelings associated with the problem. Strong feelings of dissatisfaction with the present situation often precede important changes. It is these feelings of dissatisfaction that can provide the energy or motivation for change. Personal motivation for change increases the possibility of enacting long-lasting lifestyle change. Furthermore, personal reasons for lifestyle change are much more powerful and effective than someone else's recommendations. To skip this step is to waste a valuable resource. Only after identifying the problem and its associated feelings are people actually prepared to focus on addressing the problem.

## Feelings Are Important

To a large degree, emotions and values drive all behavior. The stronger the desire to change, the stronger the investments in pursuing the identified behavior change. For this reason, it is especially important to work with the patient to help him or her identify the problem and investigate the feelings surrounding it. Appropriate solutions will arise from a strategy that values and investigates the feelings, ideals, and beliefs of the patient.

When we, as care providers in a traditional health care model, use our professional knowledge to define a patient's problem, we skip the essential first and second steps. No matter how important a provider considers a problem, it is the patient's evaluation that directs his or her priorities and actions after leaving the appointment. Excluding the patient's priorities from the problem-solving process omits the most influential player from the treatment plan. A patient's motivation for solving a problem increases when he or she considers the problem serious. The extent to which a problem is emotionally charged for the patient determines how much energy he or she will invest in solving it.

By identifying a problem and verbalizing its associated feelings, the patient gains a sense of control and an increased motivation for problem solving. It gives the patient an opportunity to untangle and clarify thinking. Addressing uncomfortable facts and expressing painful feelings, instead of denying or repressing them, increases the potential to solve the problem. Often it is not the knowledge of uncomfortable facts and the feelings that come with those facts that hurt the most, but the effort invested in avoiding their existence. Avoidance can be exhausting.

There are often two emotional aspects of the problem behavior. One is the emotional cause for excessive eating, which is part of identifying the problem. The other stems from the natural emotional resistance to behavior change. Patients will often want to know what they will have to do, what they will have to give up, and whether they can actually achieve the desired level of behavior change. Expect patients to be concerned about projected outcomes from behavior change. Often, they will want to know how the change will affect relationships, if the change will lead to the desired outcomes, and if the change will interfere with other activities. Respond to questions about expected outcomes (and refer to another professional if needed) but also be prepared to acknowledge the feelings that follow the information. Not addressing the feelings associated with an expected outcome can limit the patient's motivation for pursuing the behavior change.

## Focus on Feelings and Values

There are many possible reasons why patients may not typically
see a relationship between their feelings and/or values and
the health issues confronting them. Because this connection is
normally not seen, the patient gives less significance to behavior
change. This is why it is so important for patients and providers
to acknowledge, unearth, and understand this relationship. The
following are some reasons why unearthing this connection can
be so difficult.

- Patients are generally not used to sharing their feelings
  and/or values, especially those associated with their health
  problem.
- Patients are not used to sharing their feelings and/or values
  in a medical setting.
- Patients do not think that their feelings and/or values are
  relevant to solving the problem.
- Patients are not aware of their feelings and/or values.
- Because emotional pain can hurt, some patients place so
  much effort into avoiding their feelings or values that they
  are in fact unaware of them.
- Health care providers help patients avoid confronting their
  feelings and/or values by focusing clinic appointments on
  other issues, such as risk factors and behavior change.
- Patients may think that their care providers have to approve
  of their feelings and/or values.
- Patients often think they will be considered bad patients
  if they reveal feelings and/or values that may be judged as
  unacceptable.
- Patients may have feelings and/or values that might
  contradict a behavior change. People often fear that it is
  not appropriate to unveil such thoughts and feelings in a
  meeting on risk factors and behavior change.
- The most important problem that consumes the patient's
  energy might concern something totally unrelated to risk
  factors, weight reduction, and lifestyle change.

# Help Patients Explore and Express Feelings Associated with Their Problems

The most difficult aspect of working with the problem-solving model is addressing the patients' emotions and not trying to solve their problems for them (Anderson 1995). We seem to expect that we should solve our patient's emotional agony and often take emotional expressions, such as tears, anger, or fear, as signs of our insufficiency. Feelings are not problems to be solved. Feelings that are expressed, respected, and accepted provide "corrective emotional experiences." They enhance the patient's future ability to face threatening facts and the fear of emotional pain.

If a patient walks into your clinic and says, "I hardly eat anything at all, and I still can't lose any weight," what would you say in response? Did the patient ask a question or express an emotion? Patients express feelings and values when they feel like they are in a secure environment with an accepting, nonjudgmental health care provider. The presence of a supportive health care provider can help patients address feelings that are difficult to handle alone. Feelings are easy to ignore in a solution-centered and goal-directed health care environment.

A large part of the communication between people is nonverbal. Besides listening for words that describe feelings, information about the patient's feelings can be gathered from his or her posture, tone of voice, facial expression, and breathing, and those are just a few examples. Silence is also an important instrument for exploring feelings. It takes an average of about 3–5 seconds to formulate an answer to a question. Silence allows the patient time to reflect on a question or to recognize an insightful realization. Great things often happen in silence. If you wonder about what's going on during your patient's silence, try asking them about it.

If the patient's painful feelings have been validated, silence can lead to crying. Crying is a healthy way of releasing an emotional load. Crying does not mean that the patient needs reassurance that his or her problem is not serious or that you should try to remove the problem from discussion. Crying is a way for the patient to express feelings associated with the problem. Let the patient take his or her time while crying, and make sure that all those tears have been released. Your patient will speak when he or she is ready.

Identify explicit time limits at the beginning of an appointment. Otherwise, interrupting a crying patient by saying that his or her time is up may be perceived as punishment for crying. Explicitly formulated time limits for the meeting contribute to structure and provide the patient with some control over the session. Patients often prepare for the meeting with their health provider. Knowing the length of the meeting will allow the patient to bring up the important prepared content before the meeting is over. Offering empathy and setting boundaries both support constructive dialog.

Sometimes a patient's emotions show when he or she responds to information about illness or risk factors. These are often crisis situations for the patient. The natural course of responding to a crisis begins with shock, followed by an emotional reaction, and then concludes with working through the crisis to reorient for the future. In health care, we interfere with this process by interrupting the patient's assimilation of the information. Often, we try to provide information about the problem or try to plan for the future ahead of time. *When the patient is in shock, he or she is unable to assimilate information or plan for the future.* A health care provider's job is not only to honestly convey the seriousness of a patient's health status, but also to handle his or her personal crisis, which often follows breaking the news.

Overeating could be the result of a trauma for which the patient has not received any crisis intervention (Davis 2004, Lating 2002). If excessive eating started after a traumatic experience, offer crisis intervention, no matter how much time has passed since the traumatic experience. If the chance to acknowledge and accept a difficult or repressed experience in the past can help patients overcome excessive eating, it reduces the influence of a significant barrier to lasting weight loss.

## Questions That Help Patients Identify Feelings

- How do you feel about your weight, your eating habits, making lifestyle change, etc.?
- What are your thoughts about your weight, your eating habits, making lifestyle change, etc.?
- How will you feel if things do not change?
- Can you tell a story about this situation, including how you feel about it?

Adapted from Anderson (2005).

When asked about their feelings, patients often reply, "I don't know." In situations such as this, using silence as a tool can be helpful. Consider accepting this answer with an "OK" and a moment of silence. During this pause, the patient will sometimes open up with a flow of feelings associated with the problem behavior. For example, after being silent for a while, one patient took a pen and a piece of paper from the table and drew this (Fig. 5).

**Figure 5—A Patient Draws How She Feels**

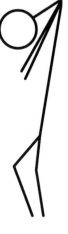

This simple stick figure communicated much about her sad feelings and the hopelessness she experienced.

To be open to hearing patients express their feelings requires that health care providers be open to their own feelings. This includes the feelings that come from listening to their patients. The experiences of patients can expose health care providers to many intense and painful stories. Emotional overload can affect the care provider's ability to empathize and lead to an emotional disassociation from the patient. Having opportunities to process and unload the feelings that come with patient interactions can help the provider remain emotionally available to identify and accept the patient's feelings. Some organizations identify mentors, colleagues, or supervisors with whom providers may discuss difficult situations without breaching patient confidence.

In the chronic-care model, all health care providers face occasions in which they will have to discuss difficult issues with their patients. Some providers are concerned that they are unprepared for this and feel that their counseling abilities are inadequate. Sometimes, they see this as an obstacle to facilitating patient self-care (Adamson 1986). However, remember that *discussing difficult issues is not the same as counseling*, which implies therapy or healing of an illness, so feeling uncomfortable at first in this situation is not necessarily a barrier to care. The kinds of interactions we are talking about do not require giving advice but instead are intended to allow patients to express their feelings and ask questions that help them clarify their situation and what they can and will do about it. The focus should be on the current situation and identifying behaviors that may improve that situation.

---

## Questions for Reflection for the Care Provider

- How do I feel when patients express positive feelings? Negative feelings?
- How do I typically respond to a patient's expression of feelings?
- What can I do to learn to calmly respond to other people's strong emotions and without judgment?

Adapted from Anderson (2005).

## Case Study 6

## Olga's Worry and Fear Subside When She Learns that She Can Get the Information and Support She Needs Over Time

Olga, 59 years old, was diagnosed with type 2 diabetes a week ago and returned for a follow-up. When asked how her week has been, Olga reported that she had responded to the emotional strain of her diagnosis by buying a cake, bringing it home, and secretly eating the whole thing. She felt like her life had been turned upside down and that her situation was unbearable. She sought further relief by having a few drinks the same night.

When asked about her feelings at the moment, Olga said that she was worried about the seriousness of diabetes and had many questions. Her aunt had diabetes and complications that affected her eyes and feet. Her aunt regularly complained about the practical difficulties of injections, blood testing, and following a rigorous diet. Olga said she anticipated major restrictions and wondered how she could ever replace the joy and relaxation she felt after treating herself with cinnamon buns and chocolate. Eating was Olga's way of coping with tough times.

Olga's husband did not have a job. She feared that the economic burden of a special diet and medical supplies would break their limited budget. When Olga was asked what she found most difficult about the diagnosis, she said that feeling like she was losing control was the hardest to accept. To her, it felt as though her life was ruled by something that she could not control. Olga also feared that she would develop the same complications as her aunt.

After a period of silence, her educator confirmed that she understood that Olga was worried. She let Olga know that her reactions were natural and that it usually took some time to adjust to the diagnosis of diabetes.

The educator also let Olga know that she would have access to the information and support she needed and suggested taking things one step at a time. Olga was given information about support groups. To make sure that Olga understood and remembered all of this new information, her care provider repeated the details about basic meal planning and the reasons for testing her blood. Olga scheduled a follow-up appointment a week later, agreed to practice testing her blood glucose levels, and made plans to write down questions she wanted answered. The educator encouraged Olga to meet with a dietitian for answers to her food-related questions and for advice about chocolate, cinnamon buns, and dietary restrictions.

## Case Study 7

### More Information Can Help Resolve an Internal Conflict

Pamela, 57 years old, participates in a weight-reduction group but has not lost any weight and does not know why. She tries and tries, but her weight remains at 202 pounds. Her situation is beginning to make her feel hopeless. However, after some discussion, Pamela realizes that she has mixed feelings about weight loss. She wants to lose weight and simultaneously fears losing weight. Pamela has leukemia and worries that weight loss will signal leukemia progression. She initially described her current situation as feeling trapped, and now she knows why. She needs more information about her leukemia before she can know whether it is safe to lose weight. She wants to know if there are signs to help her interpret whether her weight loss is a positive lifestyle change or an indicator of worsening leukemia, so she schedules an appointment with her leukemia team to get more support and information.

## Case Study 8

### Sally Recognizes Her Eating Response to Stress

Sally, 62 years old, plans to work for a few more years but feels stressed by her husband, who is retired and hard of hearing. Sally says that he shouts and nags her about everything. Sally attributes her weight problem to

*(continued)*

her frequent large serving sizes and the way she comforts herself with rolls and cakes when her husband shouts and nags. Sally's husband does not eat the pastries, but her grandchildren always ask for them at Sunday dinner, so simply cutting them from her diet would be a difficult task.

When Sally's dietitian notices that discussing the pastries and their health effects makes Sally look sad, she asks Sally how this information makes her feel. Sally says that the idea of cutting the pastries from her diet does indeed make her sad. She fears that her grandchildren will be disappointed and not come for dinner if she does not have homemade bread for them. The dietitian then asks Sally how she wants the situation to change. She responds, "I'd like it if my grandchildren brought their own bread when they visit or if they'd be satisfied not having the buns." Sally decides to discuss her problem with her daughter-in-law and ask for help. She wants to hear what her daughter-in-law might suggest. If she does not propose any solution, Sally will suggest that they bring the bread next Sunday.

At the next meeting, Sally reports full cooperation from her daughter-in-law. Now there are no tempting rolls or cakes in the house during the week. Sally is satisfied with the solution. Without rolls in the house, she has learned to cope with her husband's nagging without them. "I have accepted the situation," she says. "Now I go for a walk when I need to get away and let off some steam."

## Case Study 9
### Getting Support

Ellen is 34 years old. After her children were born (now 8 and 12 years old), Ellen never returned to her regular aerobic classes or took long walks on Sundays, so she began to gain weight. Ellen and her husband, who also gained several extra inches around his waist and had begun a diuretic for hypertension, are at risk for type 2 diabetes. Ellen's dietitian recommended that she use the rate-your-plate method to start eating healthier. By using this method, she fills one-half of her plate with nonstarchy vegetables, one-quarter with grains or starchy foods, and one-quarter with a protein-rich food. At her work cafeteria, vegetables are generously available, but at home, her husband, who prepares dinner, rarely includes them. Ellen is tired of reminding him.

Ellen does not feel supported by her family. They prefer high-fat meals, eat chips and sweets in front of the TV, and remain inactive most days. Her husband spends most of his leisure time in front of the computer. Ellen's response has been to feel angry, disappointed, sad, and lonely. She wishes she could get more support from her family to make the lifestyle changes she wants to make (and that would be good for the entire family).

Ellen decides to ask for help. She targets increasing the number of vegetables in dinner as her first behavior goal. She explains to her family that it would mean a lot to her if this symbol of healthy eating could be regularly included with the family dinner. A few weeks later, Ellen reports that her family created a way to increase the amount of vegetables at dinner. The vegetables for the week are written on the grocery list before the weekly shopping day. One family member chooses and prepares a vegetable each night. The vegetables range from raw mini carrots to fresh asparagus. This family effort was reinforced when her husband's physician recommended he see a dietitian for additional support for his hypertension. This inspired him to look for leaner versions of his usual recipes. He has found many interesting and healthy alternatives on the internet.

## Case Study 10
### Recognizing and Managing Cues to Eat

Kenneth, 69 years old, loves to eat and since retiring has done even more of it. The result is an extra 30 pounds and a second blood-pressure medication. He vividly describes how difficult it is to resist the enticing smells of food.

(continued)

Kenneth's weight gain started when he helped his neighbors put an addition onto their house. He got into the habit of eating breakfast and dinner at home but also accepted his neighbors' invitation to join them for their meals. The food smelled wonderful as he helped lay tile and hang drywall. Besides, he was getting more exercise than usual. Later, Kenneth says it was his wife's "generosity with the butter" that is responsible for those extra pounds, whereas his wife claims it was his snacking in front of TV at night that did it.

At his next physical, Kenneth became upset when he realized how much weight he had gained. Kenneth defined his problem as too much fat and high-calorie snacking at night. The dietitian helped him see ways he could reduce his fat intake and offered ideas for alternative snacks. He began to choose very-low-fat items, but at dinner simply decreased his portions because his wife wasn't willing to use less butter for cooking. To avoid the sight and smell of food that quadrupled his temptation for second helpings, he excused himself from the table after finishing his meal. Fruit was not as satisfying as a bologna sandwich while watching TV in the evening, but Kenneth got used to it. He started to lose weight and managed to maintain the weight loss. It was the information from the dietitian that got him started, but it was coming to the doctor's office for weekly weigh-ins that really helped him maintain his new eating habits. He told his doctor, "I need to come here and weigh in as a reminder of what I have done and what I need to do in the future."

## Case Study 11
### Behavior Changes Needed Even with Surgery

Alice, 53 years old, had bariatric surgery four years ago and is now regaining the weight she lost after the surgery. Alice's weight-management efforts are complicated by fibromyalgia, which limits her mobility. Her efforts are also complicated by her work as a shop assistant, which is intense and offers no regular breaks. Alice was told before surgery that the operation would help her lose weight by limiting the amount of food she could fit into her now egg-sized stomach. To benefit the most from the surgery (i.e., lose weight and improve health), the bariatric educator advised Alice to eat several small healthy meals a day. When Alice is busy at work, she never remembers to take a break for food and then becomes exceedingly hungry. She discovered that melt-in-your-mouth chocolate was easy to eat on the job and quickly satisfied her hunger without overfilling her smaller stomach. She didn't realize that it was possible to eat enough of any food to regain the weight she lost, and now she realizes that she will have to make some changes.

Alice says that she needs an opportunity to rest at work, something that she never gets. She is afraid to bother her coworkers, who always seem to be busy, and her husband does not believe that she needs any extra rest. Neither does he understand why she should require many small meals because he does just fine eating one big meal a day. A large home, a huge vegetable garden, and frequent houseguests add further demands on her leisure time. Alice is also worried that her husband does not seem to accept or acknowledge her needs. What will the future be like? She has undergone this big surgery, and now her lifestyle counteracts its results. Alice does not know where to start.

Eventually, Alice decides that her main concern is to find a way to eat regularly, as was recommended before the surgery. Alice, who has been overweight since she was a girl, begins to realize that she has tried to counteract the impression that overweight people are lazy by working harder than everyone else. Thus, her difficulty in taking breaks at work actually arose from a personal lifestyle choice. Alice discusses her situation with her boss and easily gains the support she needs to take breaks for small meals. They had the same discussion before the surgery, but now Alice is determined to change her behavior. To further support her efforts, Alice schedules an appointment with her dietitian to review the guidelines for eating after bariatric surgery. Alice also lowers her ambitions for the garden. If that doesn't relieve her exhaustion, she thinks that they could consider moving to an apartment with a balcony.

# Chapter 13

# Step Three:
# Set a Long-Term Goal

*I*n steps one and two, the patient defines the problem and explores its associated feelings. Taking step three is like crossing the bridge from defining and exploring the problem to finding a solution. Too often, we care providers skip the first two steps and jump into problem solving before the problem or what that problem means is clear. The purpose of step three is for the patient to imagine what he or she wants and to choose one or two goals that move him or her in that direction.

## Goals: Outcome and Behavior

A goal evolves from a clear definition of the problem. During steps one and two, the description of the problem might move from a vague notion of "I weigh too much" to "I weigh more than I did a year ago, which is uncomfortable because my clothes are too tight and it makes me worry that my blood pressure is up. I gained weight because I travel with my new job, which means I eat out more often and nibble food while I drive to entertain myself." A clear definition of the problem makes solving it possible.

## Visualize

If your patients want things to be better, help them picture what "better" looks like. Visualize an alternate situation to replace the current one. An often-overlooked fact is that the brain cannot visualize the absence of something. If we think about avoiding something, the brain automatically produces a picture of what we want to avoid. If we want to increase our physical activity, it will not help to think about not driving to the store. Instead, we visualize ourselves walking or biking to the store. Likewise, it will not help us to think about eating less fat. Picturing yourself eating low-fat food and many vegetables could help guide behavior toward doing so.

When I was first learning to drive, I was afraid I would hit the person coming toward me in the other lane. I intently watched the car coming toward me, trying hard to avoid it, but I didn't. I scraped the length of our door panels while driving at 3 miles per hour. My instructor said, "Keep your eyes on where you want to go, not on where you don't want to go." This lesson can be just as easily applied to behavior change.

Perceive the goal as a destination. Helping people visualize a goal is a way to support their hope and belief in the future. Introduce the idea of a functional outcome, such as feeling comfortable in certain clothing, tying your shoes, using an airplane restroom, getting down on (and up from) the floor to play with grandchildren, having reduced knee or back pain, visiting friends in a multifloor house (requires stairs), reducing the amount of diabetes medications, or taking a bike trip. One patient told me his goal was to stay well and live long enough to enjoy his retirement savings rather than to leave his money to his children.

How does this apply to people who define their ultimate goal as losing 50 pounds? What is the visual picture of that? To help visualize a goal, consider asking the patient what he or she thinks will be different when the goal weight is reached or why he or she chose that particular weight goal. Sometimes, people are told they have to lose weight and do not really know why or whether they really want to.

Formulating goals in terms of "achieving" rather than "avoiding" behavior creates a yardstick for evaluating choices. As situations and choices arise, the question becomes whether any particular action or decision will help the patient achieve his or her goal. Therefore, a patient may be able to ask, "Will eating this piece of pie help me play ball with my grandchildren next summer?" This evaluation process helps guide people toward the long-term goals they value. It also focuses effort on behavior change that improves health and well-being rather than on weight loss itself, which may or may not improve health. A clear vision of the goal helps a person reach it, even if the route changes.

# Realistic Goals

Sometimes patients' weight-reduction goals are so ambitious that they are impossible to reach (Fabricatore 2007). Our task is to explain why a particular goal may be unrealistic and to try to help patients identify goals that are more realistic. Is the goal to improve health or appearance? A large body of research has shown that total body weight reduction of 5–10 %, healthier eating habits, and increased physical activity significantly decrease health risks. Would the patient be satisfied with a weight loss of 25 pounds (10% of 250 pounds)? Would losing 25 pounds improve his or her appearance or make it easier to climb stairs? Did someone tell them they should lose 50 pounds? To facilitate success and promote health, use questions to give a patient an opportunity to identify his or her thoughts and feelings. **The challenge remains to provide information to inform choices without applying pressure to influence decisions.** If the person still settles on a goal that you think is unrealistic, accept it. In the meantime, assure your patient that he or she will learn from any effort and can always revise a goal that does not serve him or her in the long term.

# Provider Tools

For a variety of reasons, some patients are not at all sure they want to change. Take Mark, for example. Although his physician referred him to the diabetes clinic for meal planning help, Mark quickly stated he had not done what he was supposed to do in the past. Mark described himself as obese but said he accepted himself that way. He felt no great need to lose weight, even though mentally he understood that weight loss would probably improve his health. Mark did not want to put effort into achieving a goal he did not value. The fact that his brother, who was five years older, was a double amputee did not motivate or seem relevant.

The dietitian asked Mark several questions about his previous experience trying to lose weight and asked him to think about what he would like his life to be like in five years. After some thoughtful discussion, Mark realized that his blood glucose levels were seriously high, that it was important to him that he still be able to work in five years, and that lowering his blood glucose levels would increase his chances of doing so. Once he perceived a personal reason to invest in change, setting goals and developing a plan came easily.

Sometimes people need help identifying the consequences of a potential change before they can decide what to do next. Providers can guide patients through an exercise to identify the costs and benefits of making a particular change. The purpose of the exercise is not to judge a patient's evaluation but to find out how the patient values the potential consequences of his or her choice.

Motivational interviewing offers a structured way for health care staff to ask questions that help patients analyze their options (this is discussed further in chapter 16). Many patients experience a tension between their current and desired behavior. This tension makes it difficult to decide what to do. Asking the patient to rank the importance of a change for them and to estimate his or her chances of success is a way to assess his or her readiness for change.

Ambivalence might arise from low confidence in a particular approach to lifestyle change. In these cases, steps four and five in the problem-solving process will offer opportunities to try, practice, evaluate, and learn from experiments in behavior change.

## Questions to Help Patients
## Identify Long-Term Goals

- What do you want?
- How does the situation you describe need to change for you to feel better about it?
- What will you gain if you change? What will you have to give up?
- Is it worth it to you to change?
- Are you willing to take action to improve the situation?
- What needs to happen for you to get what you want?
- What do you need to do?
- Given the reality of your situation or your feelings, what can you do?

Adapted from Anderson (2005).

# Chapter 14

# Step Four: Make a Plan

S tep four creates a plan to reach the long-term goals formulated in step three. There are always several ways to reach a goal. The more possibilities identified, the greater the odds of solving the problem. Clear, vivid pictures of a goal identified in step three help generate possible ways to reach that goal.

## Brainstorm

Ask the patient to list as many behaviors as he or she can think of that might help him or her reach the long-term goal. In step four, encourage the patient to dream up options, not to evaluate the ideas. What at first appears silly or impossible may be the seed of a uniquely helpful solution.

If the patient can only think of one idea, offer some suggestions. This can be done in a collaborative, conversational way, suggesting other alternatives without trying to influence the patient's perspective. Another way to increase the number of alternative behaviors is to suggest that the patient ask his or her family and friends for ideas. Sometimes patients generate more ideas if they pretend that the long-term goal belongs to someone else who needs help finding solutions.

To model that lifestyle changes are an issue of solving problems and not an issue of following a number of rules, the health care provider should ask for the patient's opinions and suggestions and not offer any ready-made solutions. Learning a model for problem solving increases the patient's competence in dealing with problems as they arise.

The process of listing potential solutions continues until no new alternative can be found. If the scheduled time runs out before the list is complete, plan to pick up where you left off during the next appointment.

---

## Example: Brainstorming

One patient's goal of improving her eating habits consisted of two parts: 1) to distribute food throughout the day by eating three evenly spaced meals with two planned snacks and 2) to improve the quality of her food intake by including vegetables at dinner. She brainstormed the following list of potential behaviors:

- stop working
- leave work earlier
- have snacks
- have a fruit on the way home from work
- prepare vegetables for dinner in the morning
- drink water during the day
- make a weekly menu (meal plan)
- plan next day's meals the night before
- ask her husband to bring food home every night
- order take-out food every night
- replace dinner with a low-calorie frozen meal
- eat out a lot

Clearly, some of these ideas will not help the patient achieve her goals, but the role of brainstorming is to simply get ideas out of the mind and into discussion. During brainstorming, don't discourage the patient in his or her efforts. Instead, save discussion for later, when both the patient and provider can collaboratively determine a strategy for making the goal a reality.

# Prioritize

Next, the patient chooses one behavior from the list to try. Small behavior-change steps that fit into established routines with little disruption increase the possibility of success.

The patient uses these three steps to narrow the list:

1. Remove any behaviors from the list that are unappealing or impractical to the patient.
2. Rank the remaining behaviors. Ease and benefit are typically the deciding factors.
3. Choose one or two of the highest ranked items to develop a plan.

---

## Example: Ranking Options

This is how the patient in the example on page 122 valued her options. Notice that the range can be arbitrary. This patient chose a value of 1 to 7 for simplicity and because the other options were not appealing to her. In her range, 1 is the most promising option and 7 is the least promising option.

- ~~stop working~~
- ~~leave work earlier~~
- have snacks (rank 4)
- have a fruit on the way home from work (rank 2)
- prepare vegetables for dinner in the morning (rank 7)
- drink water during the day (rank 3)
- make a weekly menu (meal plan) (rank 5)
- plan next day's meals the night before (rank 1)
- ask my husband to bring food home every night (rank 6)
- ~~order take-out food every night~~
- ~~replace dinner with a low-calorie frozen meal~~
- ~~eat out a lot~~

# Make a Specific Action Plan

The action plan provides the nuts and bolts of problem solving. After all of the thinking, talking, and feeling, the action plan details the specific things the patient will **do** to solve the problem. This step is critical, yet problem solving is one of the least addressed behavior goals in diabetes education programs (Zgibor 2007). Problem solving requires much teaching and coaching in the beginning. To help develop a clear action plan, address the following questions:

1. What to do
2. How much to do it
3. When to do it
4. How often to do it
5. When to start

If the patient is having difficulty developing an action plan, try rephrasing or clarifying the action plan to make sure the patient knows what he or she specifically has to do. Action planning is a skill that improves with practice and experience.

---

### Example: Action Plan

The patient in the previous example decided that planning menus ahead of time was the best strategy for meeting her goal of eating satisfying meals with more nutrients and fewer calories. She decided to begin by planning menus for just the evening meal. This is the action plan she created.

| | |
|---|---|
| 1. What to do: | Plan tomorrow's menu and see if anything has to be purchased or prepared in advance. |
| 2. How much to do it: | Focus on the evening meal |
| 3. When to do it: | After dinner, before cleaning up the kitchen. |
| 4. How often to do it: | Sunday through Thursday. |
| 5. When to start: | This coming Sunday. |

Providing a secure environment in which to experiment with new behaviors is a critical component of this step. If the patient anticipates judgment or any form of subtle punishment from less-than-perfect execution of the plan, the potential for learning and ultimate success is diminished. As is emphasized in step 5, there are no mistakes or failures in a problem-solving process; instead, there are only opportunities to learn from efforts in behavior change.

---

### Questions to Help Patients Identify a Plan

- What are some ideas you have about strategies that might work?
- What have you tried in the past?
- Why do you think that did or didn't work?
- What are some steps you could take to bring you closer to where you want to be?
- What do you need to do to get started?
- Is there one thing that you can do when you leave here to improve things for yourself?

Adapted from Anderson (2005).

---

## SMART Goals

Using the SMART model (Top Achievement 2011) can also be helpful in guiding patients to develop their own goals. Each letter in SMART identifies a characteristic of realistic, achievable goals, helping people get the most results out of their goal development (Table 9).

**Table 9—Using the SMART System**

|   | Characteristic | Think about... | Example |
|---|---|---|---|
| S | Specific | What do I plan to **do**? What action will I take? Can I describe this action clearly enough that someone else could do the same thing? | Walk for exercise. |
| M | Measurable | How will I know I am making progress and when I have reached my goal? | Walk for 10 minutes per day for 3 days per week. I will write how many minutes I walk each day on my calendar. |
| A | Attainable | Do I have the resources (time, money, energy, space, ability) to do this activity? | I will set out my clothes the night before and be dressed before breakfast. Then I will be ready to walk soon after the kids leave for school. |
| R | Realistic | Given all my other commitments, is this activity a priority? What will I have to give up to make time for this? | It is very important that I start to move more. Ten minutes isn't much exercise, but it is a realistic start for me. I will have to give up my second cup of coffee after the kids leave. |
| T | Timely | Is this a good time to start the activity? | The kids are in school and the weather is still nice, so now is a start time that will work. |

## Case Study 12
### Identifying Choices

Robyn, 34 years old, and her husband, Andrew, would like to start a family, but Robyn realizes that the 40 pounds she gained after marriage may interfere with her ability to conceive. Robyn and Andrew appreciate a fine meal and enjoy eating together. Andrew is very athletic, whereas

Robyn sometimes eats for comfort when life gets rough. She loves cheese and could easily finish 3–4 ounces before dinner.

Robyn trusts her husband's love and does not believe losing weight would change their relationship. However, the extra weight causes other problems. Robyn believes her weight causes others to treat her disrespectfully. Right in front of her, Robyn's in-laws often make insulting remarks about her size. She tries to laugh but feels angry and sad. One night, Andrew's thin and physically fit former girlfriend ran into them in a restaurant and sat down at their table for a while. The woman ignored Robyn the entire time, as if she did not exist. Contrary to what people may think when they see her, Robyn does care about her appearance but finds it difficult to find attractive styles in her size.

Robyn evaluates the dietary habits that contribute to her excess weight. Recognizing her tendency to overeat when she skips a meal, her long-term goal is to eat meals on a regular basis. For support, she joined a weight-reduction group at the health care center. She appreciates sharing experiences with other participants. This is how she describes her experience with the group: "Some of them have thicker skins than I do, and it is good to see somebody who refuses to feel belittled because she is overweight." This group has helped Robyn realize that she does not have to accept blame or be ashamed of her weight. "I know that I am overweight, and I am dealing with that," she tells us.

Robyn enjoys physical activity and knows it would help manage her weight, but she does not want to attend another gym class alone. She feels exposed and hates to undress in front of others in the locker room. She resolves her dilemma by recruiting someone in her weight-reduction group to join her in a gym class for larger people. Robyn also learns how to read food labels to help her evaluate eating options. "I know that I can choose to have an afternoon treat, but that it will add calories," she says. "It is a choice I have to make."

## Case Study 13
### Planning for New Options

Betty, 34 years old, lived in another part of the country until four years ago, when she met a man on an internet dating site and moved across the country to live with him. Betty has gained almost 50 pounds so far, with no end in sight. Betty cries when she describes her situation and has difficulty defining her main problem. Her relationship with the man did not turn out as she wished. His need for his mother's approval has a much higher priority than his relationship with Betty. He also objects to her outgoing nature when she wants to go out with her friends.

Betty has started to regret her move but cannot return now. She would not be able to get a job due to the strong prejudices against obese people in her former community. "I have always taken care of everybody else and now I can't even take care of myself," she cried. "I just eat all the time." Betty's struggle with her weight was not new, but her experiences with losing weight and regaining the lost weight never included anything like her current weight gain. Betty misses her family but is afraid of visiting her parents because of her weight gain. She also misses her brother, but the last time they met, he told her to get gastric surgery. Betty wants to change her eating pattern on her own.

Betty has a full schedule. She works in a nursing home. She enjoys working with patients, but worries that her aching back and the pain in her knees and feet may soon prevent her from doing her job. Betty works irregular shifts, which interferes with her goal to eat regularly. In hopes of moving to an administrative position at the nursing home with fewer physical demands, Betty takes clerical classes at night. She also gives weekly classes in bridge, competes in bridge tournaments, and has close friends among the bridge players.

Betty defines her problems as her unlimited eating, her relationship with this man, an overbooked calendar, and no time to relax. She decides to first focus on her eating habits and agrees to keep a food record for four days before our next meeting.

Her food record reflected her irregular work schedule. Because of her night classes, Betty often ate dinner late, and by then her appetite was huge. She also stays up late because she describes herself as a night person. She does her homework late at night. In addition, Betty suffers from insomnia, so she's tired in the mornings. She often skips breakfast to arrive at work on time. Some days, she has lunch at her job. Betty developed the habit of eating leftovers from her patients' plates rather than returning them to the kitchen, where she knew workers would throw it away. Betty finds it difficult to waste food, but by skipping breakfast and sometimes lunch, Betty became more susceptible to eating her patients' leftover food.

Betty worked to improve her eating habits during the following months. She stopped cleaning up the patients' food, reminding herself it was not her responsibility to avoid wasting food. She met with a dietitian to develop a realistic meal plan. Although she continued her relationship with her boyfriend, Betty moved into her own apartment. They are now on a friendlier basis than when they were living together, and she can see the positive traits that drew her to move here.

Betty accepts the fact that she has a weight problem and will always need to pay attention to maintaining a regular eating routine. Very recently, she started an administrative job at the nursing home with steady hours. Having completed the night courses, she has time to meet friends, play bridge, and relax. Betty says that she moved here too quickly. She might move back some day but plans to stay for now. Her relatives come to visit, and she goes to see them.

## Case Study 14
### Coping Options

Beatrice, 32 years old, gained weight following a muscular disease that left her physically disabled. She is married and has a part-time job. *(continued)*

She follows her recommended meal plan to avoid weight gain but has difficulty resisting sweets.

Bea is used to responsibility and calculating the consequences of her actions. "I know if I physically overdo it, I pay with pain," she told me. Her toughest challenge is limiting sweets. "If I resolve to avoid all sweets, I can get angry, sad, and easily irritated by my husband and colleagues," she said. "It's just easier to eat the sweets."

Bea's goal is to continue losing weight and to get rid of her craving for sweets. She recognized that special situations trigger the craving, particularly conflicts with her colleagues and her husband. She observed, "I can bear the conflicts with my colleagues, but with my husband, they never seem to end."

One year later, Bea and her husband filed for divorce. They were unable to resolve their conflict. Bea was unwilling to keep eating sweets to cope with the conflict, and she had not found a healthier alternative. "I have come to understand that I will be better off on my own than together with him," she said at her latest visit.

## Case Study 15
### Planning Specifics

John, 56 years old, is a widower. He is short and muscular beneath his excess adipose tissue (BMI >40 kg/m$^2$). John began to gain weight after leaving a physically demanding job for a desk job.

John learned at his recent checkup that he had developed hypertension and high cholesterol. John asked if there was anything he could do to get rid of those problems. The educator talked with John for a while and told him that making healthier food choices and including more activity could lower his risks, but she could not promise that the problems would disappear. When John realized how much risk was attributed to his weight, he became determined to change his lifestyle. Fortunately, other than a "bad knee," obesity had not interfered with his ability to be active.

John decided he would limit any behavior changes to weekdays. He has met a woman who means a lot to him, and he values their weekends together. He enjoys their relaxing meals and does not want to put pressure on her to make changes that she has not initiated herself. To lower his calories, John decided to cut back on his fat intake. He learned that he could tolerate chicken and fish more often and eased up on the salad dressing and bedtime peanuts. He also doubled his usual serving of vegetables, but without the butter. He began walking 30 minutes during lunchtime and compensated for that time by working 30 minutes later.

John wanted to be in control. He found an internet program that could calculate his caloric needs and add up the calories he took in each day. He calculated the number of calories he needed each day in order to lose about a pound a week. John calls for an appointment when he feels he needs one. Two months later, John scheduled an appointment. He was pleased with the progress he had made by integrating some changes into his usual schedule and had found it easier than he expected. His friend Molly supports his lifestyle changes, as do his colleagues and boss.

# Make Another Plan

Good planning includes preparing for obstacles. The risk of relapse decreases when one discusses and prepares for potential obstacles. Thus, one of the provider's tasks is to help the patient anticipate and prevent any practical or emotional obstacle that might interfere with implementing the plan.

If we do not encourage patients to anticipate obstacles, we leave them stranded with disappointment. How many people succeed with a new behavior from the very beginning? Not addressing obstacles implies that there is no risk of obstacles appearing. Avoiding discussion of obstacles also suggests that it is the patient's fault if they arise. From experience, we know the value of assessing obstacles and of having more than one plan. To enhance the chances of success, we can help patients develop not only a Plan A, but also a Plan B, C, and D for implementing behavior change.

Preparing for obstacles is a way to expand a patient's realm of security. It counteracts "black or white" and "win or lose" styles of thinking. The attitude marked by "black or white" thinking contributes to the common problem in which any temporary lapse to an old behavior is viewed as a sign of failure rather than as a learning opportunity. Encouraging alternative solutions to a problem behavior emphasizes that there is no last chance in the problem-solving process. The process continues until the problem is solved.

## Questions to Help Patients Identify Obstacles

- What could prevent you from succeeding in this plan?
- What personal attitudes, feelings, or thoughts do you think may prevent you from succeeding?
- Are there any people or common situations in your daily environment that may stop you from reaching your goal?
- Are there any situations that could prevent you from fulfilling what you have planned?

Changes in mood may interfere with adherence to a behavior change plan. Different states of mind arouse different behaviors. An action plan that is carefully planned and easily executed when one is calm and relaxed may not be as easily executed or seem as carefully planned when the same person is upset or stressed. Patients can sometimes plan for such events by using sticky notes, alarms, planners, or other methods to recall the plan when their minds are elsewhere. One patient bought a ring to help recall her strategy in stressful situations. The ring reminds her of her goal and that sticking with her planned snacks is a way to make the goal come true.

## Case Study 16
### Violet Speaks Up

Violet, 27 years old, is a customer service representative in a technical office, but she feels insecure in that role. She cannot keep up with the constant flow of new information and therefore cannot answer many of the questions customers ask. Her colleagues seem to give her a lot of work, and she is afraid to decline because she does not want to anger them. Violet keeps a smile on her face and says that she has always functioned like that. As a girl, she tried to please her parents, who she believes did not like her. She wants others to like her and often says "yes" when she means "no," even when friends ask for money or to spend the night in her convenient downtown apartment.

On the way home from work, Violet often stops at the grocery store for comfort food: chips, bread, cookies, other snacks, and beer. She seldom buys fruits or vegetables. When she gets home, she opens a can of beer as she walks inside the door. Then food, TV, and magazines provide relaxation until bedtime.

Violet defines her main problem as her job. She does not want to work there. She wants to become an artist, but she has to support herself in the meantime. Violet's ultimate goal is to enjoy work and not feel tense all the time. Her long-term goals are to feel more self-confident when her customers call and to be able to say no to her colleagues when they pile work on her desk. Violet brainstormed the following list of possible action plans and ranked them.

- Talk to her boss about her situation (rank 1)
- Create routines for updating her technical competence (rank 3)
- Find someone to mentor her at work (rank 2)
- Plan spare time each day for important and stressful issues (rank 4)

Violet prioritized her options and decided to speak with her boss first. If her boss could not address the problem, then Violet created a Plan B. Plan B was to call her human resources department and ask for counseling. Violet decided to ask her boss for a meeting the next morning. If her boss was not there, Violet would write him a letter.

## Case Study 17
## Party Survival for Catherine

Catherine, 39 years old, participates in a lifestyle support group. One of her long-term goals is to eat nutritious meals on a regular schedule. Catherine enjoys food and is unable to store any tempting food in her refrigerator without eating every bite. Frozen food does not tempt her, but anything with flavor threatens her meal plan.

Catherine plans to host a dinner party for her friends and begins to prepare for the challenging situation to follow. What will she do with the leftovers? Her experience is that she finishes all of the leftovers herself right after the guests leave, during the night, or before noon the next day. She always feels miserable afterward, but cannot stop herself from finishing all of it. Catherine needs a strategy for solving her problem and asks her support group for ideas. After a collective brainstorming of solutions ranging from throwing the food away to freezing it, Catherine decides to pack small boxes with the leftovers and give these to her guests when they leave. Her Plan B is to give it to her neighbors, a young family with three children. Her Plan C is to throw away the food. Catherine wishes that she could keep the food but is realistic about it. In her current situation, she needs to get the food out of her flat; otherwise it hinders the behavior she values. A month later, Catherine tells her group that she packed small plastic boxes with leftovers for the guests to take home, which they appreciated. Once she found a plan that worked, she did not fear having company.

## Case Study 18
## Not Now

Annette, 27 years old, has a BMI of 32 kg/m$^2$ and a waist circumference of 56 inches. So far, she has none of the risk factors often associated with obesity, is self-confident, and enjoys a good relationship with her husband. Annette is aware and concerned about her increased risk for type 2 diabetes because her mother has it. Annette recently gained some weight that she attributes to excessive eating for emotional reasons due to turbulence at her job. Annette went to a health care center with a friend to participate in a weight-loss group.

Annette kept a food diary for a week that reflected healthy eating most of the time. After that exercise, Annette realized she was not prepared to eat less or to make any other changes right then. "I really do not feel like working on this right now," she told us, "but I am afraid I will become like my mother and not have the power to lose weight or change my lifestyle." Because she had no current medical problems and her job situation that prompted the excess eating was resolving, Annette decided not to actively work toward weight loss at this time. She did decide to evaluate her risk factors regularly, so she would know if her health was at risk. Annette decided that she could muster the necessary motivation if her health depended on it.

## Case Study 19
### Steve's Travel Plans

Steve, 45 years old, suffers from sleep apnea. He tried an acrylic splint and continuous positive airway pressure (CPAP) without success before he learned that excess weight substantially contributed to his sleep apnea.

Steve's sleep apnea bothered him and his wife so much that Steve decided to lose weight and resolved to change his habits. He listed many possible ways to improve his food choices and quickly integrated some of them into his lifestyle. When Steve and his wife planned a trip to visit her family for a week, they discussed how they might handle Steve's food concerns during their stay.

Steve expressed his concern and said, "Dinner is their only meal, and *(continued)* beyond that, there are no limits. During the day, everybody eats whatever he or she wants whenever they want. No one in the family cares for vegetables. To be extreme, they might include a tomato. I am used to eating half a plate of vegetables every night. More than that, I need to eat three meals a day and probably a snack or two to stay on track." His wife supported Steve's interest in maintaining his new habits without offending her parents. She agreed to join him for breakfast and lunch and to talk to her mother about Steve's health concerns and the reasons why they wanted to eat on a schedule. They would also offer to provide vegetables every night and keep canned fruits and vegetables in their trunk to supplement available food if needed.

## Case Study 20
### More Water

Jennifer, 49 years old, is married and works full time at a construction office. Her two sons have left home. Jennifer is neither conscious of when she is hungry nor when she is satisfied. "I forget to eat during the day, and at night I eat until the pots and pans are empty." Because one of her sons has diabetes, Jennifer learned to plan healthy, well-balanced meals and continued to do so after her sons left home. It is the timing and portions of meals that cause problems. Jennifer realizes that her excess weight affects her well-being. "I do not feel well," she said. "My stress at work interferes with my eating, but I am afraid I will get sick if I continue like this."

Jennifer decided to begin eating breakfast every day and to moderate her portions. She also planned to drink six cups of water every day. Jennifer remembered feeling better when she used to drink more water, perhaps because it seemed to ease her problems with constipation. When Jennifer next met with her support group, she reported doing well eating breakfast every day but could not get started drinking water. She asked the group to brainstorm ideas to help her drink more water. This is how her list looked when she had prioritized the alternatives.

- Buy five big bottles of water from a nearby grocery store every Friday during lunch. Put one bottle on her desk every morning and finish it before going home (rank 1)
- Get a nice water pitcher and glass to put on her desk
- Program her watch alarm to beep every hour to remind her to drink (rank 3)
- Every time she reaches for the calendar, take a sip of water
- Reward herself for drinking water by getting a magazine on Friday, when she buys the water (rank 2)
- Recycle the empty bottles and donate the proceeds to charity
- Save the lids in a container and watch it fill up

Her Plan B is that if she has not finished today's bottle when it is time to leave work, she brings the bottle home. Jennifer is satisfied with these solutions and will start on Friday, when she will get the water supply for next week.

# Chapter 15

# Step Five:
# Evaluate the Result

*T*he aim of step five is to evaluate what did and did not work. Did the behavior changes, planned in step four, work well in practice? Whether they worked well or not, this is the time to plan what happens next and continue the problem-solving process (Fig. 6).

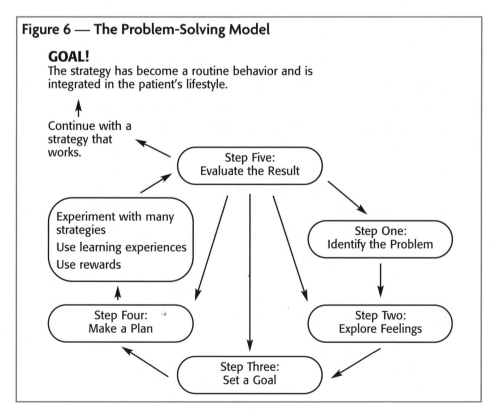

**Figure 6 — The Problem-Solving Model**

**GOAL!**
The strategy has become a routine behavior and is integrated in the patient's lifestyle.

Continue with a strategy that works.

Step Five:
Evaluate the Result

Experiment with many strategies
Use learning experiences
Use rewards

Step One:
Identify the Problem

Step Four:
Make a Plan

Step Two:
Explore Feelings

Step Three:
Set a Goal

# Why?

Problem solving is an ongoing process that involves exploring problems, planning changes, and trying different solutions. This process would not be complete without a time to evaluate whether the chosen efforts worked in bringing the patient closer to his or her goals.

When sailing, we take our bearings, adjust our sails to the wind, and chart our course in order to reach our destination. This same process is true for behavior change. Patients identify obstacles and decide how to handle them. They regularly have to take their bearings to see if their plan is feasible, acceptable, and effective. As we evaluate our efforts, it becomes evident that behavior change is a process and not a single action.

# When?

Consistent with the collaborative problem-solving process, the patient decides when to schedule his or her next appointment with the health care provider. Typically, when patients begin the problem-solving process, every week or every other week is the preferred frequency. If patients come less often, they can easily lose focus. Later in the process, patients might join a support group for more frequent contact in order to supplement the less frequent individual appointments with the health care team. Some patients prefer to schedule the next appointment for evaluation as they plan the strategy. Others prefer time to try out their planned changes before they call for follow-up.

We encourage patients to evaluate their own solutions. This takes time. One patient carried a small pad to write down notes on new insights about herself while experimenting with new behaviors. Try asking patients how much time they have available for personal follow-up, reflection, and planning. When in the day might that happen? The exercise in Fig. 7 may be useful in helping patients plan.

## Figure 7—How I Spend My Time

**I.** Use this figure to illustrate how you spend your time. One activity could fill many segments and one segment could be filled with several activities.

Think about activities like these:

1. Household chores
2. Work
3. Reading, studying
4. Physical activity
5. Sleep
6. Meeting with friends
7. Transportation
8. Watch TV
9. Relaxing
10. . . . . . . . . . . . . . . . . . . . . .
11. . . . . . . . . . . . . . . . . . . . . .
12. . . . . . . . . . . . . . . . . . . . . .
13. . . . . . . . . . . . . . . . . . . . . .
14. . . . . . . . . . . . . . . . . . . . . .

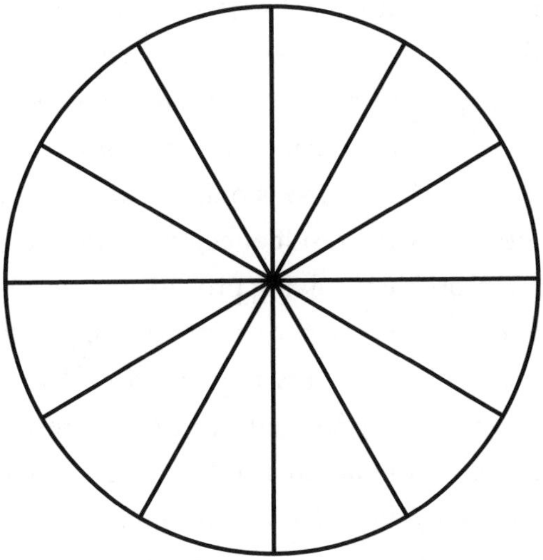

**II.** Consider when you will reflect on and evaluate your strategies for reaching your goals and your priorities for how you will spend your time.

1. Household chores
2. Work
3. Reading, studying
4. Physical activity
5. Sleep
6. Meeting with friends
7. Transportation
8. Watch TV
9. Relaxing
10. Reflecting on strategy
11. . . . . . . . . . . . . . . . . . . . . .
12. . . . . . . . . . . . . . . . . . . . . .
13. . . . . . . . . . . . . . . . . . . . . .
14. . . . . . . . . . . . . . . . . . . . . .

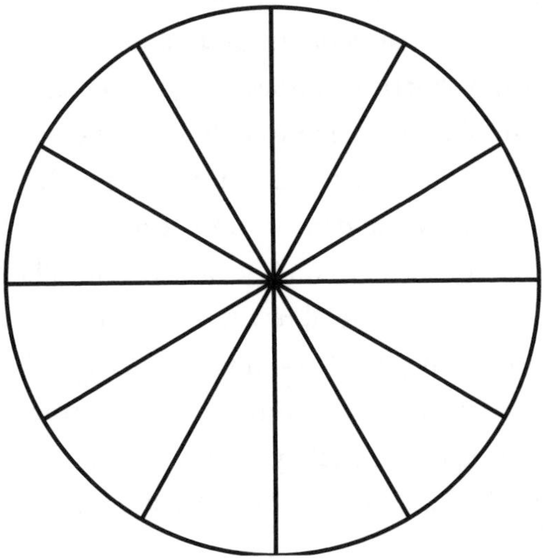

# How?

Our task is to support patients' efforts to achieve the behavior change they have chosen. We therefore provide patients with a secure environment for behavior experiments and reflection. A secure environment requires that we neither praise nor blame patients for their actions or for the result. Praising is a way of saying that we are in a position to judge the patient. Expectations that a health care provider will judge the results of their experiments inhibit patients' efforts to attempt new solutions. The health care provider's opinion of the result does not matter. What matters is how the result affects patients and their problem-solving capacities.

A problem-solving process is an expedition into unexplored territory. Every step is a sign of courage and worthy of respect. A secure environment offers patients the chance to learn the way adults learn best—by experimenting and reflecting on the results. A nonjudgmental way to help patients evaluate their efforts and support insights might be to ask them what they did, what they thought of the process, and how it made them feel. This approach to evaluation supports patients' problem-solving capacity and affirms the benefits from every experiment.

This approach of listening to, acknowledging, and helping patients learn from their experiments is quite different from judging the performance or outcome of the behavior itself. It counteracts an all-or-nothing attitude that is often found among obese people. With this model, even if the experiment does not turn out as expected or hoped, it still provides useful information to help solve the problem.

If the patient finds this perspective difficult to grasp, suggest other examples that demonstrate learning as a process of trial and error. Home repair programs on TV rarely show all of the mistakes, missteps, and trials before the final result is achieved. Athletes are not followed during the endless hours of training; we just see their physical achievements during a brief display. Encourage patients to consider disappointments as learning experiences; they are opportunities to better understand and solve the problem. If they become frustrated by slow progress, try asking patients if they allow enough time to learn new things. Do they expect everything to run smoothly from the beginning? Do they have any role model for problem solving? Questions facilitate the learning process. When patients have not reached their goals, we should ask them why not or what obstacles prevented them from reaching their goals. The answers to such questions will help patients uncover behavior options that can help them progress toward their goals.

There are some patients who seem to continuously plan lifestyle changes but never accomplish them. Many reasons may contribute to an indifferent attitude toward problem solving. We do not help patients by joining in their casual attitude. Instead, we help by probing their understanding of and attitude toward their risk factors and challenging their priorities.

There are occasions when patients achieve their long-term behavior goals and reduce metabolic risk factors without achieving the planned weight loss. When asked to explain the reasons and expectations for the first two, patients often revise their initial weight goals and settle for the more reasonable and achievable target. Such discussions can bring closure and help patients come to peace with their weight outcomes.

---

## Questions to Help Patients Reflect on Behavior Change Experiments

- What did you learn as a result of setting this goal?
- What did you learn as you attempted to achieve this goal?
- What would you do differently next time? What would you do the same?
- What barriers did you encounter? What ideas do you have for strategies to overcome those barriers?
- How do you feel about what you accomplished?
- Were you able to do more or less than you thought you would be able to do? Why? (If the patient is unable to do as much as expected, ask the following questions.) Do you think that the problem was with the long-term goal or with the

*(continued)*

strategy? Is this still an area on which you want to work?
- What did you learn about yourself as a result of this experiment?
- Did you learn things about the kind of support you have, want, or need?
- What did you learn about how you feel about this problem or area of change?
- What did you learn about how valuable or important this goal is to you?

Adapted from Anderson (2005).

# Chapter 16

# Useful Models
# and Methods

*"There are more things in heaven and earth, Horatio,*
*than are dreamt of in your philosophy."*
—Shakespeare, Hamlet (I, v, 166–167)

Beth has gained 40 pounds over the last 15 years. At a recent physical, her doctor explained how the weight gain and family history increased her risk for type 2 diabetes. Her doctor associated these risks with Beth's present eating pattern. Beth became concerned about her health, so she decided to lose weight and reduce her risks. For about six months, Beth successfully lost about 15 pounds, but then slowly returned to her former eating habits and regained the lost weight.

Health care providers often expect their patients to behave in a way that improves their health. This does not always happen. Why? Because the care provider does not consider the problem from the patient's perspective. We must acknowledge that behavior change is difficult to institute and maintain for the patient (or any individual). The best way to understand what does and does not work for a patient will be to understand the foundations of his or her life. The box below shows the complex matrix of values, feelings, attitudes, lifestyle preferences, social environment, and patient-provider interactions that influence the perception of a proposed behavior change.

## The Patient's Perspective

A person is more likely to change if he or she...
- identifies personal benefits associated with the change and believes it will improve his or her well-being and quality of life.
- feels an internal motivation and that the behavior change is a result of his or her own free choice.
- believes that he or she can do it, feels safe, and has positive expectations.
- understands the problem and how it can be solved.
- gets social and professional support and knows that others believe in his or her success.
- sees others succeed and realizes that if these goals are possible for others, then they are equally possible for the patient.

A person is less likely to change if he or she...
- values the present lifestyle more than a lifestyle change.
- experiences strong external pressure for behavior change.
- doubts his or her power to accomplish a satisfying result.
- feels insecure, has negative expectations, and worries about problems regarding the change.
- is stressed and his or her acute problems take a lot of energy and attention.

Pressure to change interferes with the patient's ability to make real changes. Real changes are authentic and consistent with the person's beliefs, priorities, and interests. Most of us have made changes to please others, whether for parents, teachers, bosses, or health care providers. But if these changes don't fit, the person living with the changes will feel uncomfortable and be at high risk for recidivism. It is difficult for health care professionals who treat obesity to avoid projecting their values onto their patients, but it is in the best interests for both parties.

We may be used to saying things that imply pressure even when we are trying to remain neutral. Table 10 offers some examples of "value-loaded" phrases and possible alternatives.

## Table 10—Watch Your Words

| Typical Statement | Consider |
| --- | --- |
| "You should eat breakfast." | "Research shows that people who eat breakfast burn more of their total calories and are less likely to develop insulin resistance." |
| "You shouldn't eat candy." | "Candy provides many calories per bite and offers few nutrients that help your body take care of you. When you eat candy, it is harder to get the nutrients you need without eating more calories than your body can use." |
| "Take this medicine once a day to help you lose weight." | "This medicine keeps you from digesting all of the fat you eat and allows it to pass through without absorbing the calories it contains. If you eat too much fat, the side effects of the medicine become obvious and will make you uncomfortable." |
| "Hmm, not enough progress. Time to schedule you with a dietitian." | "A dietitian can be a resource who will help you find different ways to adjust your eating habits and lower your calorie intake." |
| "You have to lose weight." | "Your weight has gone up since I last saw you. Your blood pressure is up as well, so I will need to recommend increasing your blood pressure medication. How ready are you to talk about weight loss as a way to lower your blood pressure?" |
| "You have to keep a food record." | "Food records tell you about yourself. If you are aware of what you are eating, then you have more power to change. The more information you record, the more you can learn." <br><br> *Note*: Some providers make keeping food records a requirement for working with them. Yet, everyone still has a choice of whether working with that professional is worth the requirement. |
| "Join a weight-loss program." | "It may be helpful if you join a weight-management or lifestyle program. Are you interested in this? Let's discuss what options might work best with your personality and lifestyle." |

# The Health Belief Model

The Health Belief Model (Strecher 1986, Rosenstock 1988) offers additional insight into factors that affect health behavior. It describes a person's health-related behavior as a function of how he or she experiences four key areas: 1) the severity of risk factors, 2) personal susceptibility and vulnerability to complications, 3) the benefits of and obstacles to following health recommendations, and 4) his or her self-efficacy.

## Severity of Risk Factors

Obesity—and especially central or abdominal obesity—is a risk factor for type 2 diabetes and other components of the metabolic syndrome. A society that values thinness as a cosmetic issue blurs the focus on obesity as a health risk. To focus attention on obesity as a health issue, Kushner (2005) recommends that primary care follow-ups regularly address BMI, waist circumference, and other metabolic risk factors and offer support for a lifestyle change.

## Personal Susceptibility and Vulnerability to Complications

Information about risk factors does not automatically cause individuals to see themselves as facing a risky situation (see Case Study 4 in chapter 11). Denial is a psychological defense that can block the association of metabolic risk factors with personal vulnerability. The onset of medical problems, such as diagnosis of type 2 diabetes, knee pain, or heart failure, may serve as a wake-up call and prompt health-related behavior change. Losing a friend or relative to the complications of these conditions can also highlight susceptibility and trigger action.

## Benefits of and Obstacles to Following Health Recommendations

Behavior is motivated by the needs it meets. Patients behave in a way that satisfies their own prioritized needs. Making a sustained lifestyle change is not just a question of adding new behaviors to the usual repertoire, such as taking medication or following a prescribed diet for a limited time. Changing also implies removing old habits, which may function well in meeting other personal needs. Established behaviors may maintain a sense of well-being, even though they also contribute to obesity. Other obligations may override someone's intent to improve an eating habit.

---

## Case Study 21
### Redefining the Problem

When Beth returned to her health care provider after regaining weight, she explained how the only comfort and relaxation in her stressful life came from her usual eating habits. Furthermore, she didn't have the time to plan meals. Her obligations to her children and her job had to be met before she could think about changing her eating habits.

Given this situation, what is Beth's next step? Using the problem-solving model is a great way to help people identify realistic changes. By solving problems, patients will be able to determine whether the benefits of a change (i.e., improved health, more energy, weight loss) exceed the costs of a change (i.e., time, effort, and inconvenience).

Beth defined her primary problem as her stressful daily life. She needed more time in her daily schedule, so she decided to use the car for shopping and for driving the children to different activities instead of using the bus. She decided to use that extra time for meal planning. Because of this decision, Beth was able to purchase the ingredients she needed by shopping twice a week rather than running to the store every day. Three nights a week, she began walking at the sports center while her children swam. After another year, Beth found a less stressful job. She explained that these small changes gave her space to breathe, something she vitally needed in order to successfully change her eating habits. Subsequently, she lost weight and gained more energy to invest in further improving her self-care habits.

# Self-Efficacy

Self-efficacy is a person's confidence in his or her ability to change a specific behavior. It is considered a key factor in successful behavior change (Bandura 1977). An individual's self-efficacy varies across situations. An emotional overeater might feel very confident about resisting the temptation to overeat at work, but less so when socializing or needing emotional comfort. Repeated experiences with losing and regaining weight decrease a patient's self-efficacy for making sustained eating behavior changes. Experiences with successful behavior change strengthen self-efficacy and provide the necessary confidence to tackle further change. It follows that even goals with no measurable clinical benefit (e.g., walking for five minutes three days a week) can be a significant step toward improved health. Appropriate role models can aid self-efficacy. Patients observing others succeed in accomplishing relevant behavior changes can improve their own self-efficacy (Bandura 2001).

The next section offers more practical tools that facilitate rapport between patient and provider and foster a mutual understanding of the situation.

# Readiness for Change

The Health Belief Model can increase our insight into complex problems. As discussed earlier in this book, obesity may result from many and various internal and external factors. Regardless of those factors, the motivation for a behavior change relates directly to the personal meaning that change has for the patient. Motivation provides the energy for the task and must come from the person making the change.

In assessing an individual's readiness for change, Rollnick (1999) suggests a way to quickly evaluate the extent to which someone values a behavior change. Two questions measure the importance the patient attributes to the change and his or her confidence in making the change (i.e., self-efficacy). Many educators use the following questions to assess readiness.

## Question 1: Importance

Assess importance by asking this question:
"On a scale from 0 to 10, with 0 being the least and
10 the most, how important is it for you to
_____(insert specific change)_____?"

Not
Important    0 – 1 – 2 – 3 – 4 – 5 – 6 – 7 – 8 – 9 – 10    Very
Important

For example, Beth rates her plan to eat breakfast an "8" in importance. When asked some clarifying questions, she explains that it is more important to her to eat breakfast than to empty the dishwasher or sweep the kitchen floor. She is willing to face those tasks when she gets home from work. Preparing breakfast for her children and getting to work on time, however, are more important than eating breakfast herself.

## Question 2: Confidence

Find out about a patient's confidence by asking this question:
"On a scale from 0 to 10, with 0 being the least and
10 the most, how likely are you to succeed with
_____(insert specific change)_____?"

Not
Likely    0 – 1 – 2 – 3 – 4 – 5 – 6 – 7 – 8 – 9 – 10    Very
Likely

Beth estimates her confidence in eating breakfast every day as a "4." She lists several obstacles to success. Many things interfere with her efforts to get to work on time. She mentions how hard it is to get up in the morning, the competition for the bathroom, the time it takes to fix her hair, her husband's last-minute ironing requests, her dislike for typical breakfast foods, and her boss's extreme insistence on punctuality.

Success in achieving goals is more likely when a person's confidence and importance ratings are greater than 7 (Gooley 2005). If confidence is rated at 7 or lower, ask what it would take to increase confidence. Perhaps an easier goal or enlisting support will increase the confidence level and the likelihood that the goal will be accomplished. Sometimes, small changes require big effort.

Beth decided to modify her goal from eating breakfast every day to eating breakfast twice a week. She found peanut butter on toast and juice to be an acceptable quick breakfast. If time was tight, she planned to drink an instant breakfast on the way to work and kept breakfast bars in her work desk as further backup. Success at eating breakfast twice a week is likely to build Beth's confidence toward eventually reaching her primary goal.

## Cost as a Barrier

In addition to the insurance concern, many valued lifestyle changes come with some financial costs. There is often an initial investment in exercise equipment. Walking shoes, a pedometer, a new bathing suit, or membership at a fitness club are not free. Fresh fruits and vegetables, ground sirloin, and whole-grain bread are more expensive than potato chips, regular ground beef, and white bread. Some neighborhoods cannot support a grocery store, which can limit access to fresh and unprocessed foods.

Unemployment, economic changes, and competing financial priorities may interfere with one's ability to pay for the extras required for behavior change. Many patients feel ashamed of their financial problems and hesitate to reveal them as obstacles to behavior change.

If someone's waning energy to achieve goals does relate to financial concerns, he or she is usually relieved when a team member addresses the issue directly. He or she may appreciate the opportunity to hear about lower-cost options and to learn whether economic support is available. This discussion may also be the time to identify inexpensive rewards for reinforcing progress in behavior change.

## Time Outs

Successful lifestyle change does not imply continuous effort or improvement. A stressful life situation, lack of family support, and economic problems are frequent barriers to behavior change and often prompt patients to drop out of a program. Other concerns may become more important and limit the time and energy available to work on personal behavior changes. Countless temporary situations demand our attention for a time: family illness, visiting in-laws, holidays, relationship crises, vacations, moving, a flooded basement, and youth sport playoffs are just a few examples. Allowing other needs to temporarily assume priority does not mean quitting lifestyle change efforts. Perhaps during these particularly busy periods, one can maintain some but not all of their usual efforts, such as including breakfast but giving up the aerobics class when hosting houseguests. If someone is taking part in a formal program, simply continuing to attend may help maintain progress and offer a sense of continuity in a stressful situation. When other situations are no longer a major concern, people can resume their behavior change efforts. Others may need to modify their goals.

# Motivational Interviewing

Our patients' attitudes, beliefs, and values have more influence over their behavior than knowledge, and we cannot change them (Anderson 2005). However, we can help them reflect on those attitudes, beliefs, and values and the associated consequences and decide whether they support or impede the accomplishment of their desired goals. Motivational interviewing (Miller 2002) details techniques that stimulate personal reflection and enhance intrinsic motivation for change. It is a nonconfrontational counseling tool consistent with the collaborative relationship between patients and providers described in this book. There are four principles that characterize motivational interviewing: *1)* express empathy, *2)* develop discrepancies, *3)* roll with resistance, and *4)* support self-efficacy.

# Express Empathy

This principle is designed to help the provider understand how the patient experiences the problem. Emotional needs, rather than the need for physical energy (i.e., calories), often motivate excess eating. If a patient tries a weight-reduction strategy that interferes with the way he or she usually satisfies emotional needs (i.e., often emotional eating), then conflict appears. Such a conflict can affect the patient's well-being and may block the behavior change effort if it goes unaddressed. It is the health care provider's responsibility to accept the validity of the patient's needs that currently motivate his or her behavior.

Expressing empathy does not mean just being sympathetic or kind to someone with a problem. Using empathy requires that the care provider try to understand and associate with the patient's experiences and requires intense listening. In short, our listening guides the questions we ask.

---

## Some Ways to Express Empathy

- Ask open-ended questions that cannot be answered with a simple yes or no. For example, asking how something makes the patient feel will facilitate a broader answer than simply asking, "Did this make you feel sad?"
- Listen carefully, not just to the spoken words but also to the tone and body language. The quality of your listening communicates your level of respect for and interest in the patient's experience.
- Summarize and rephrase what the patient says without interrupting with opinions or suggestions. This confirms the authenticity of your interest and provides an opportunity to correct possible misunderstandings. The patient may clarify and/or discover contradictions in his or her way of thinking. This process often leads the patient to a better understanding of him- or herself and encourages further sharing.

## Develop Discrepancies

Developing discrepancies highlights gaps between the patient's present status or situation and his or her expressed goals and values. This principle is intended to help the patient see the gap without judgment. Becoming aware of the gap taps into the energy that drives change.

---

### Case Study 22
### Mona Sees a Discrepancy

Mona's goal was to increase her physical activity. She planned to walk every day between 5:30 and 6:00 p.m. after work. She discussed this with her health care provider.

"What day will you start your plan?" her health care provider asked.

"Next week," Mona said, but in an absent-minded way.

"Okay, and on what specific day do you want to begin?"

"I'm not sure," Mona answered. "Tuesday?"

"And on what days are your son's soccer games?" her provider asked. There was silence while Mona stopped to think.

Then, laughing, she exclaimed, "What was I thinking? I can't walk every night!" Mona concluded that walking three nights a week (on Mondays, Wednesdays, and Thursdays) would be more realistic given her other commitments. She would buy new walking shoes during the weekend and start the following Monday.

---

## Roll with Resistance

Many patients resist health care recommendations, but the care provider must avoid confrontation or arguments designed to change patients' point of view. When advocating lifestyle change, you cannot expect the patient's point of view to ever change. The more successful alternative is to roll with resistance.

Patients express their resistance in a variety of ways. Some arrive at their visit angry, hostile, or confrontational and not at all pleased with being there.

Patients may be angry about a new diagnosis, upset with the care he or she has received, concerned about missing work to be at the visit, annoyed with the neighbor's dog, or grieving over a recent death. Some arrive after reading a book or scouring the internet and make it clear that they have already decided on their treatment plan. *Their behavior is not about you, but your response will influence subsequent interactions between you and the patient.* Therefore, arguing with a patient or trying to change a patient's preconceptions interferes with accomplishing the goals of the current visit. However, this approach does not require that you agree with the patient's ideas when you don't. Honesty is a key component of the chronic-care approach.

Being chronically late, frequently canceling appointments, or just not showing up at all can be an expression of resistance. Patients are communicating that their current plan is not effective. It may be that they don't believe the appointment will be worth the time and money to get there, but they are unable to tell you this directly. The challenge for the provider is to uncover the patient's reasons for avoiding appointments.

The possible reasons for resistance are endless. Perhaps the planned change brings out other issues that have yet to be addressed. For example, skipping an evening snack may upset a cherished household routine. Any behavior, including old habits and new behavior changes, has positive and negative consequences. Perhaps the planned change requires more time than planned, such as the time required to get to the gym as well as the workout time. Perhaps the patient verbally agreed to eat breakfast, but did not agree to schedule the extra time required to actually eat that breakfast. Perhaps something in the patient's daily life has changed, such as losing a job or being promoted to a more demanding position. Return to empathetic listening and develop discrepancies to help the patient uncover his or her barriers.

## Support Self-Efficacy

As discussed earlier, self-efficacy is a person's confidence that he or she can successfully make a change. Successful small changes increase patient self-efficacy and support further efforts for change. For this reason, the problem-solving model that helps patients identify realistic and achievable goals now sets the stage for successful behavior change in the years ahead.

The importance of supporting self-efficacy is one reason why behavior change rather than weight loss defines short-term goals. Weight is the consequence of behavior change, but changes in body weight do not accurately reflect behavior change. Weight loss can occur for multiple reasons, some healthy and others not. Scale weight can vary from one day to the next as a result of constipation or fluid retention, providing unpredictable and transitory measures of success. Tracking behavior change keeps the patient in control of his or her success and makes it possible to build self-efficacy.

In addition, a single behavior change may not measurably affect scale weight but is a necessary step to reaching a long-term goal. For example, an obese patient who does not exercise begins to increase physical activity by using the treadmill for five minutes a day. It is unlikely that after a week any objective measure can assess the progress toward a long-term goal. Choosing a treadmill, figuring out where to put it, buying appropriate shoes, and actually walking five minutes a day requires significant effort and are necessary building blocks for further change. Repeatedly setting, reaching, and acknowledging small changes builds self-efficacy and cumulatively restructures the lifestyle habits that influence body weight over the long term.

# Social Support

Social support is an important and well-known facilitator for achieving a behavior change. Maintaining a lifelong effort to change habits and lose weight is a challenging long-term project with many opportunities to lose focus. Support can be viewed as what people need to refuel and keep going. It recharges rather than drains their batteries.

Although everyone benefits from support at one time or another, what constitutes support is extremely individual. Some need practical support and others emotional support. Some need structure, whereas others resent it. Some gain energy from diversions, helping other people, or just listening to birds sing. Ask patients where they get support and what they need or think would help them. Table 11 offers some suggestions that can be helpful if the patient requests support (Green Pastors 2003).

## Table 11—Possible Sources of Support

| Interactions | Personal time | Stimulation | Activity |
|---|---|---|---|
| family | massage | theater | travel |
| friends | yoga | music | watching nature |
| phone calls | counseling | movies | hiking |
| support groups | spiritual practice | television | exercise |
| coworkers | reflection | internet | playing sports |
| professional groups | solitude | reading | redecorating |
| volunteer groups | keeping a journal | workshops | cleaning a closet |
| helping others | hobbies | work | gardening |

Adapted from Green Pastors (2003).

Although they may not feel comfortable at first, encourage people to assertively ask for what they need. Those who are able to identify and use their support sources can expand their capacity for making positive behavior changes.

## Some More Questions

These additional questions (Feste 1992) may help people identify potential support.

- What does support mean to you?
- Where can you get support?
- What obstacles might prevent you from getting the support you need?
- Do the people who support you know what kind of support you need?
- Are you putting up barriers that prevent others from supporting you?
- How do you encourage others to support you?

People who have psychological issues with food, are depressed, or have other emotional or mental obstacles might require professional help to address these barriers to lifestyle change.

# Stress and Coping

If a stressful life situation and insufficient coping are obstructing behavior change, consider posing these questions (Feste 1992).

- What are your primary sources of stress?
- Is the stressor a problem? Is it a problem that can be solved? Reflect on how you might solve it.
- How do you cope with stress? In what ways are your coping choices good for you? Do you feel that they are successful? To what extent?

If your coping strategies are not as successful as you'd like, how might you improve them?

# Ambivalence

There is both a benefit and a cost to every behavior change. Whether the benefit is worth the cost is sometimes unclear. When the pros and cons are unclear, ambivalence is often the result. Ambivalence does not drive change; it stalls change. Ambivalence is normal, but it can be the most difficult phase in the behavior change process.

Table 12 illustrates an example of one strategy to help patients clarify the pros and cons of a behavior change. Divide a box into four sections with room to list the costs and benefits of making and not making a change. Help the patient identify the emotional as well as practical consequences of a change.

## Table 12—Evaluate Your Options

Proposed behavior change: Walk up the stairs three times a day

| If I Change | If I Don't Change |
|---|---|
| **Positive** | **Positive** |
| • Reduced metabolic risk factors (long term) | • My usual habits are more comfortable and require less work (short term) |
| • Weight loss (long term) | |
| • More self-confidence (long term) | • I could continue with my job and let the job take the time it needs without interruption (short term) |
| • Better able to walk without getting out of breath (long term) | |
| • Increased chances of living longer (long term) | • I won't raise others' expectations and risk disappointing them (short term) |
| • Less knee pain (long term) | • I don't have to explain my actions to my colleagues (short term) |
| **Negative** | **Negative** |
| • Takes time to walk up the stairs (short term) | • Risk of myocardial infarction/heart attack (long term) |
| • Interrupts the work day (short term) | • Risk of stroke (long term) |
| • Have to tell others about my decision and face their reaction (short term) | • Risk of type 2 diabetes (long term) |
| • I have tried so many times before without succeeding, and I am afraid of failing again (long term) | • Risk of impaired mobility due to joint problems (long term) |

When the grid is complete, help him or her look for patterns. Are the short-term benefits perceived as more valuable than the long-term benefits from a behavior change? Are short-term behavior changes too difficult to be worth the effort? The resistance toward change increases in parallel with the amount that the change will affect daily routines, meal habits, and physical activity. This exercise might result in the patient making short-term goals easier to achieve and self-rewards more frequent.

A scale reads the same whether one loses five pounds by drinking meal replacements or by increasing fruits and vegetables while limiting after-dinner snacks. The first is probably easier and faster, but it is not sustainable. The second is probably more difficult and takes longer, but it invests in long-term health. If health is the long-term goal, a system that reinforces positive behavior change, not pounds lost, makes much more sense.

Ambivalence is a significant barrier to behavior change, and helping patients look more closely at their preferred outcomes helps them overcome ambivalence and continue with healthy progress. Apart from using a decisional balance sheet for assessing ambivalence, ask other questions to address readiness for change and identify competing needs or other obstacles to change.

## More Questions for Addressing Ambivalence

- What do you gain if you don't address this problem?
- If you solve the problem, what do you gain?
- Where do you want to be in one year?
- What happens if you do not do anything now?

Adapted from Anderson (2005).

## Case Study 23
### Ian Weighs the Pros and Cons

Ian, 53 years old, is an administrative executive. He has abdominal obesity and other risk factors for hypertension. Ian's job is stressful, and he has nonexistent physical activity patterns. His knees have started to ache. He defines his long-term goal as reducing his risk factors by increasing his physical activity. Ian regularly comes to his appointments but does not make the behavior changes he plans. His latest short-term goal was to take the elevator to the basement and walk up the stairs to his office three times a day. However, he has not done it yet. His health care provider wonders how Ian perceives the costs and benefits of his proposed behavior change. She describes the cost-benefit exercise, and Ian agrees to complete a chart to help sort out his options.

*(continued)*

The results of Ian's worksheet (Table 12) show that his desired long-term benefits favor a behavior change and that the short-term benefits do not. When asked to rate the importance of his walks, Ian gives it a "7." Ian actually attributes more value to this behavior change and to his health than his colleagues might think or appreciate. He considers achieving these health-related goals more important than his duties to his job. However, it was only after seeing it on paper that Ian realized that this lifestyle change was in fact very important to him.

When asked about where he would be in a year if he did not lower his risk factors, he mentions his granddaughter and talks about his special long-term project at work. He recognizes that not following through on his action plan may jeopardize his future plans. He decides that the life and health benefits of increased exercise are worth the effort. Instead of making one more phone call, he will use the time he scheduled for it to take a walk. If there is a meeting during his scheduled walk time, he will suggest a short break.

Ian considers himself a role model for his fellow colleagues. He is not the only man with central obesity and metabolic risk factors at his company. Ian mentions that he could benefit from changing his eating habits. However, his wife is not open to any changes right now, and he will need support. Ian schedules a follow-up appointment in two weeks. Until then, he will observe his eating habits and consider possible improvements.

# Chapter 17

# Practical Information

*I*n chapter 3, we described the fundamental lifestyle issues that influence obesity: food choices, cravings, and activity level. People regularly receive information on lifestyle issues and health behaviors, but few (30%) reflect on the personal meaning of the information and consider whether there are reasons to change their own behavior (Kegan 1994, Kjellström 2005). Millions of Americans remain practically illiterate about health issues to the extent that they have trouble reading a prescription label. The average American is unable to access, understand, or use available information to help them make healthful food choices (US Department of Health and Human Service 2008).

## Food Habits

The basics of healthy eating (i.e., eating a variety of whole grains, fresh fruits, vegetables, lean protein, lean dairy products, and small amounts of unsaturated fat) are readily available and generally apply to people trying to lose weight. Translating these guidelines into actual meals is more challenging.

Too often, people unnecessarily restrict food or eat things they do not like because they heard it was "good for them." Myths surrounding eating and obesity abound, fueling false conceptions, and creating an eager market for quick-fix diets. Referral to a dietitian or other qualified dietary professional for assessment of individual needs and accurate information can prevent useless efforts and sometimes dangerous consequences. Expert advice is especially valuable for those with other chronic medical problems who want recommendations integrated into one meal plan. For further explanation of dietary guidelines, help with meal planning, and referral information, see the Resources section.

Assuming that a patient has an accurate and appropriate meal plan, the primary problems in learning to eat well are establishing new routines, solving practical problems, and changing a pattern of emotional eating (Anderson 2005, Kegan 1994, Adolfsson 2002, Sarlio-Lähteenkorva 1998, Perri 2001). The following sections identify sample situations that make establishing new routines difficult and suggest possible alternate behaviors. Listen for these and other risky situations in your patients' stories. Being aware of situations that can undermine goals can be a step toward reducing the strength of those risks.

## Table 13—Food Habits

| Risky Eating Behavior | Reason Why Behavior Is Risky | Alternate Behavior Options |
|---|---|---|
| Irregular meal times | More calories are used when evenly distributed throughout the day | Eat every 4–5 hours or have a planned snack |
| Skipping meals | Skipping breakfast is a risk factor for insulin resistance | |
| | Risk for excess hunger and overeating | |
| Unaware of caloric and nutritional content of food | Can't make informed choices without information | Learn what is in food, e.g., which types of foods are high in carbohydrate, protein, fat, and calories |
| | | Use food labels |

| Risky Eating Behavior | Reason Why Behavior Is Risky | Alternate Behavior Options |
|---|---|---|
| Eating out often | Food is almost always higher in calories and sodium than similar foods prepared at home | Eat out less often |
| | | Order plain food |
| | | Eat less. Share portions |
| | Lack of available information about nutrients in restaurant food | Use resources to learn more |
| | Menu descriptions do not tell how food was prepared | Ask questions |
| Not having food available that supports desired goals (this happens to people who don't shop, shop without a list, or shop when hungry) | Can't eat what is not available, so they: | |
| | • Eat out more often | Shop regularly |
| | • Buy inappropriate food | Purchase only foods that fit into the meal plan |
| | • Buy more than they need | Shop when not hungry |
| | (Once high-calorie food is in the house, it will be eaten) | |
| Unplanned snacking | Excess caloric intake | Plan and carry appropriate snacks |
| | | Substitute lower-calorie snacks, e.g., an apple instead of beer and chips while watching TV |
| Mindless eating: Eating automatically because it is associated with another activity such as having a snack when cooking or having beer and chips when relaxing in front of the TV | Excess caloric intake | Notice hunger |
| | | Evaluate nutritional quality and serving size of the snack |

| Risky Eating Behavior | Reason Why Behavior Is Risky | Alternate Behavior Options |
|---|---|---|
| Eating quickly | Excess caloric intake | Plan at least 20 minutes to eat |
| | It takes 20 minutes for your stomach to let your brain know that you are full | |
| | Fast eating is a form of mindless eating; not experiencing eating increases the risk of eating more | Notice and enjoy food |
| | Indigestion | Chew well, which increases surface area for digestive enzymes and stimulates saliva production |
| Believing false messages, such as "eat this and still be slim" | Friends, family, coworkers, and advertising offer reams of misleading and sometimes dangerous information | Be critical! Use your own knowledge and common sense to evaluate information on food and diets |
| | Anything that promises to make weight loss quicker or easier can be tempting but is possibly unhealthy | Seek information that is based in science and is practical |
| Difficulty leaving food on the plate (family value to not waste food) | Excess caloric intake | Consider which is more wasteful, extra food in the garbage or around your waist |
| Social events, holidays, etc. | Excess caloric intake | Plan for these (see Resources) |
| Eating without a plan | No basis for decision making | Tailored dietetic guidelines decrease cravings and unplanned snacking |
| | Unplanned snacking | |
| Reliance on "tried and true" family recipes | Unknown nutritional content of foods | Learn to adjust "old" recipes into healthier ones |

# Craving: Where It Comes From

A craving (or "faulty" hunger awareness) is an urge to eat that is not related to physiological hunger. Learning the difference between physiological and psychological hunger may take time, especially for those who do not remember experiencing true hunger. Eating in response to psychological hunger cues creates a high risk for excess calories. Even the best meal plans will not satisfy psychological cravings. It is far more proactive to help the patient identify and address the source of these cravings than to help them override or ignore their cravings.

Chapter 3 described several forms of craving in order to illustrate the many complex factors that contribute to obesity. We think it is helpful to appreciate the power of cravings that drive hunger. Use the lists that follow to increase awareness of these cravings, how they might present, and the possible approaches to reduce their influence. The problem-solving model is built on listening to the issues the patient raises and on asking questions to help patients clarify their statements. Suggestions to schedule empty time for reflection or seek ways to laugh are helpful approaches to dealing with the stress that may emerge from problem solving. Avoiding uncomfortable topics does not serve the needs of the patient; however, assuming the role of a therapist in treating mental disorders is also beyond the scope of practice for most health educators. For treatment of problems such as posttraumatic stress syndrome or sexual abuse issues, refer patients to a counseling professional. Obviously, if patients reveal situations that put them or others in danger, then promptly contact a professional qualified to address such concerns.

## *Stress*

Stress is almost universal, but responses to stress vary. Many people manage stress with food, making weight management more difficult. There may be realistic options for reducing stress; but for many people, learning new coping strategies is a critical step in the weight-reduction process (Table 14).

## Table 14—Stress and Its Sources

| Risky Situation | Tips for Active, Problem-Focused Methods of Coping with Stress |
| --- | --- |
| • Stress overload, with no time for relaxation<br>• Lack of time to reflect and regain balance<br>• Insufficient coping strategies<br>• Interrupted routines<br>• Sudden changes with no time to prepare<br>• Conflict<br>• Expectations perceived as too difficult or impossible to meet<br>• Major life changes that may be happy or sad, e.g., birth, marriage, divorce, death, buying a house, child leaving home, moving, etc. | • Regular and healthy dietary habits protect from stress overload<br>• Social support is a protective factor in times of stress—ask for support<br>• Physical activity is effective in counteracting the negative consequences of stress<br>• Schedule "empty" or leisure time for reflection and relaxation on a calendar<br>• Laughing helps to distance oneself from the situation and produces endorphins, a hormone that soothes pain and increases well-being<br>• Identify early signals of stress overload and break an escalating stress spiral before it happens<br>• Identify the stressor<br>• Learn effective coping strategies<br>• Vacations can help defuse stress |

## *External Stimuli*

Research suggests that obese people are more sensitive to external stimuli compared with normal-weight people. Therefore, routine situations may precipitate cravings and excess eating in sensitive people (Table 15).

## Table 15—Situations that Offer Patients Either Too Few or Too Many Stimuli

| Risky Situation | Tips to Avoid Overeating in Response to External Stimuli or Boredom |
|---|---|
| • Any environment that presents more stimuli than the patient can process (e.g., grocery store, heavy traffic, cafeteria)<br>• Occasions that increase external cues to eat (e.g., vacation, holidays, social gatherings, advertising)<br>• Situations that increase monotony (or boredom) (e.g., unemployment, retirement, sick leave, structured/quick-fix diets with repetitive meals) | • Establish routines for healthy dietary management<br>• Get support from significant others to follow dietary routines<br>• Increase awareness of surroundings; prepare for risky situations, reflect on what could happen, and create an emotional readiness for what to do<br>• Find non-eating ways to cope with boredom<br>• Find new activities to reduce boredom<br>• Become familiar with and accept routines; seek alternative sources of stimulation; increase awareness of surroundings |

### *Sleep and Fatigue*

Unsatisfactory sleep and fatigue may induce overeating, too (Table 16).

## Table 16—Unsatisfactory Sleep and Fatigue

| Risky Situation | Tips to Reduce Fatigue |
|---|---|
| • Insufficient sleep and rest<br>• Difficulty saying no to external and internal demands increases the risk of stress overload | • Get a sufficient amount of sleep<br>• Learn to prioritize personal needs<br>• Get support from significant others<br>• Increase body awareness |

### *Anxiety*

Anxiety and other painful feelings often cause cravings (Table 17).

**Table 17—Anxiety and Other Painful Feelings**

| Risky Situation | Tips for Coping with These Painful Feelings |
|---|---|
| • All situations in which painful feelings are soothed or avoided by eating | • Notice how physiological hunger feels<br>• Pay attention to hunger cues. Are they physiological or emotional states?<br>• Become conscious of and verbalize the inner conflict that causes anxiety (verbalizing increases control and decreases the need for excessive eating that compensates for insufficient psychological defenses)<br>• Seek a health care provider or support group with whom it is safe to express the feelings otherwise soothed by eating |

### *Trauma*

Excessive eating can be a symptom of untreated traumatic experiences (Davis 2003, Lating 2002). The excessive eating defends against painful memories and releases tension associated with the trauma. If eating and obesity function to repress traumatic memories, underlying problems are likely to emerge when eating patterns change. Because the delayed impact of traumatic experience can derail efforts to change eating habits, evaluation for insufficiently or untreated trauma may be an important screening variable. Successful resolution of posttraumatic symptoms may be a prerequisite for successful weight-loss efforts. Unresolved trauma increases sensitivity to later traumas and other stressors (Table 18).

## Table 18—Unresolved Trauma

| Risky Situation | Tips to Resolve Symptoms of Trauma |
|---|---|
| • History of traumatic experience (e.g., war, death, fire, flood, sexual abuse) | • Refer to a qualified professional to discuss traumatic experiences<br>• Especially helpful to learn effective coping strategies for stress to avoid an eating response |

### *Sexual Difficulties*

Addressing sexual difficulty depends on many factors, including its extent, the provider's level of knowledge and comfort, and the patient-provider relationship. In some cases, concerns about sexual difficulty can be addressed with various members of the health care team, whereas some patients may be better served if they are appropriately referred (Table 19).

## Table 19—Sexual Difficulties

| Risky Situation | Approaches to Dealing with Sexual Difficulties* |
|---|---|
| • Problems with sexual identification<br>• History of traumatic sexual experiences<br>• Disturbances in current relationship with partner<br>• Becoming single | • Provide information<br>• Debrief sexual trauma<br>• Involve partner in lifestyle change<br>• Attend a support group<br>• Become secure with sexual identity<br>• Accept sexual impulses and, when necessary, learn to control them<br>• Increase body awareness |

*A counseling professional's expertise may be appropriate in order to accomplish some options.

### *Group Expectations*

The expectations of others can influence behavior change (Table 20).

**Table 20—Group Expectations**

| Risky Situation | Tips to Buffer Expectations from Others |
|---|---|
| • Lack of support for lifestyle change from family members and from other significant people | • Involve family and significant others in lifestyle change activities<br>• Join a support group |

# Physical Activity

This is not a book on physical activity. Support from an exercise specialist may be necessary to identify appropriate activities for an obese person. It is unrealistic and unkind to ask a person who suffers from functional impairment and chronic pain to walk for 30 minutes. Even if the ultimate goal is a 30-minute walk, the first step might be to stretch the arms above the head or to rise from sitting or lying on the floor to an upright position.

## What Is the Patient Thinking?

The following list illustrates the kinds of questions obese patients will often ask while preparing to increase their physical activity.

- How hard do you need to exercise to feel good and maintain weight loss?
- Does jogging for 30 minutes burn more calories than walking for the same amount of time?
- Do two periods of physical activity of 15 minutes each equal a single 30-minute session?
- What is the easiest way to burn fat?
- Does spinning hurt your back?
- Is water aerobics good exercise?
- What physical activity is easy on the knees?
- What physical activity can you recommend for losing weight without risking injury?

What information, support, and guidance might your patients need to safely and effectively exercise? Obesity itself creates additional challenges to exercise; yet exercise is a key ingredient in improving and coping with obesity-related problems.

## Table 21—Situations and Conditions that Discourage Activity

| Risky Situation | Tips to Encourage Movement |
|---|---|
| • Physical limitations (e.g., arthritis, back problems, Charcot foot) <br>• Fatigue <br>• Exercise is disliked <br>• A vicious circle of decreased physical activity and increased obesity, which prevents physical activity <br>• Overcommitted schedule <br>• Travel <br>• House guests <br>• Poor access to workout locations | • Try new modes of activity that are safe and possible given current physical ability (water aerobics and Nordic walking are two examples of physical activity appreciated by overweight and obese people) <br>• Ask for help from an exercise specialist or work with a trainer to identify appropriate activities |

# Chapter 18

# Maintenance

$S$uccessful long-term weight loss is defined as an intentional 10% weight reduction from baseline that is maintained for one year (Wing 2005). Weight loss is usually concentrated during the first three to six months of the program (Korner 2003) and regained within five years (Byrne 2003, NIH Technology Assessment Conference Panel 1992, Cooper 2003, McGuire 1999).

## Why Maintenance?

Most weight-reduction programs focus on the weight-loss period and target weight loss only. Weight reduction is not synonymous with achieving a healthier lifestyle and sustained weight control. Often the weight loss is regained in three years. If weight reduction is maintained for up to five years, then the chances for long-term success greatly increase (Byrne 2003). Among people succeeding with sustained weight loss, some behaviors have been common, including healthier dietary habits and increased physical activity—behaviors that have also been reported to promote a decrease in metabolic risk factors. The WHO (2007) underlines the importance of an ongoing weight-maintenance program after the weight loss has been achieved and emphasizes that successful long-term weight maintenance depends on continuing follow-up.

Setting a time restriction of a few months and excluding maintenance from a weight-reduction program have two major negative consequences.

First, it implies that weight maintenance is an easy, do-it-yourself task; otherwise, it would have been included in the program. Second, excluding a weight-maintenance period does not teach participants how to integrate their new behaviors into their lifestyles. Acquiring new habits, which could last a lifetime without impairing quality of life, requires these habits to fit into the patient's lifestyle. Without closing the gap between following a restricted diet for weight loss and adapting to healthy eating in everyday life, the patient will naturally regain weight after the program ends. To help a patient plan for lifelong weight management, consider the following issues.

# Learn the Difference between Weight Reduction and Weight Maintenance

Achieving temporary weight loss is different from achieving sustained weight maintenance (Hill 2005). A patient's main problem in achieving weight maintenance is not ignorance of healthy eating or of the health benefits from physical activity; rather it is an issue of establishing new routines, solving practical problems, and changing a pattern of emotional eating (Anderson 2005, Kegan 1994, Adolfsson 2002, Sarlio-Lähteenkorva 1998, Perri 2001). Prochaska (1995) reports that at any one time, only 20% of patients are ready and therefore successful in actively changing behavior. Prochaska, Norcross, and DiClemente (1995) found in a representative sample across more than 15 high-risk behaviors that less than 20% of a problem population is prepared for an active behavior change at any given time. In order to increase the chances for a sustained behavior change, a motivational phase that included an emotional arousal connected to the problem behavior needed to be focused before the action took place.

Patients' difficulty in maintaining new behaviors is seldom reported in the media. Instead, happy weight-losers show off their new outfits and stunning transformations as proof of the effectiveness of a certain weight-reduction program or crash diet before behavior changes have been fully integrated into their lives. Expecting weight maintenance from a patient without including it in the weight-reduction program is like expecting somebody to perform the lead part in *Swan Lake* by giving them a pair of ballet shoes but no training. It is like planning a big fancy wedding but not addressing the changes that come with being married.

The challenge to maintain weight is greater than the challenge to lose weight. How often have you heard a colleague remark that if a drug had the long-term success rate of weight-loss programs, they would never have made it to the pharmacy?

## Clues from Research

Newer studies offer glimmers of hope and clues to long-term maintenance. After four years, AHEAD participants in the intensive lifestyle intervention group have sustained 6% weight loss (and reduced their need for medications) (The Look AHEAD Research Group 2010).

The Diabetes Prevention Program (DPP, NIH 2008) documented that small amounts of weight loss make a difference. In this study, a modest reduction in weight (5–7%) with diet and exercise (150 minutes per week) substantially (58%) lowered the rate of diabetes for obese subjects with prediabetes. That means weight loss of 10–20 pounds for those starting at 150–250 pounds improved their **overall health**. Perhaps if the primary goal is health, then this realistic target can be less overwhelming and success more likely than setting a goal to reach some "ideal weight" or fit into a certain clothing size.

The National Weight Control Registry (www.nwcr.ws) has now collected more than 5,000 stories of people who have maintained an average loss of 66 pounds for 5.5 years. Success stories come from a diverse group of people, who report having lost weight using a variety of strategies, with (55%) and without (45%) the help of some type of program. The unifying trait is a strong commitment to maintenance.

Walden (2004) reports that weight control programs lasting 16–26 weeks can be sustained with continued patient-therapist contact. Because ongoing professional support is likely to become cost prohibitive, self-help programs as a follow-up to more intensive behavior modification treatment offer another viable option for supporting long-term maintenance (Latner 2001). Self-help groups are voluntary and based on equal values and mutuality among the members in the group. In such groups, transforming those who have received help into the providers of help has not only been found to increase the resources exponentially, it has also meant positive consequences for the provider (Reissman 1990). Providing care to others offers the former patient a more active role and the chance to feel less dependent, more giving, more socially competent, and more open to learning in order to teach others.

# Teach Problem Solving from the Beginning

Different models for including the maintenance phase in weight-reduction activities have been tried. No consistent results are yet available. However, one distinction has become apparent between those who are able and those who are unable to maintain changes. Those able to maintain a behavior change were those who learned to problem solve from the beginning of treatment.

One of the authors of this book conducted a lifestyle intervention program for obese participants. The program began with lifestyle seminars that met for 12 consecutive weeks at 90 minutes each. The seminars offered the problem-solving model described in this book. To ensure participants received accurate and adequate information with which to make informed choices, a physiotherapist addressed physical activity and a dietitian covered eating habits and dietetic questions in four additional sessions. Consistent with the content of the seminars, participants received written materials for review and engaged in physical activity at a nearby fitness institute at least three times a week.

Relationships among group participants grew during the presentation weeks and continued as they transitioned into a self-help group that met weekly for another six months. The seminar presenter attended the first three weeks to help the group learn to function as a support group. During these small group sessions, most participants sustained their positive changes, and some succeeded in further weight loss.

When using the problem-solving model, the patient's short-term behavior goals are integrated into his or her everyday life. Problem solving becomes a habit for the patient and not another new skill to learn for maintaining weight loss. When the behavioral approaches to weight loss suggested by this book are applied, there is little difference between the strategies for weight loss and weight maintenance. This chapter reiterates concepts discussed elsewhere to illustrate why.

# Focus on Behavior Instead of Weight

WHO states that the worldwide increase in obesity is due to lifestyle issues, i.e., changes in eating habits and levels of physical activity. Population studies show that losing 3–5% of total body weight, incorporating healthy eating habits, and increasing physical activity levels decrease the prevalence of type 2 diabetes by between 30 and 60% among patients with impaired glucose tolerance (Tuomilehto 2001, Knowler 2002). That lifestyle issues affect cardiovascular disease risk was confirmed in a longitudinal survey of 22,000 American men (Lee 1999). In this study, there was no difference in cardiovascular morbidity / mortality between physically active men of normal and excess weight. However, exercise made such a difference that even inactive normal-weight men were at a higher risk for cardiovascular disease than physically active obese men. Although genetic and medical factors contribute to these risk factors, the recent explosion in weight gain is not due to evolution but to behavior patterns. Individuals have no power over their genetics but do have the potential to change behavior patterns.

Stegemann (2011) states that obesity is a chronic disease and cannot be cured, even with surgery. Providing ongoing education and follow-up in a setting where patients feel comfortable enough to report lapses supports patient efforts for long-term weight maintenance.

Even though lifestyle and behavior are targets for change, weight loss programs typically use a scale to measure progress. Yet, weight loss and improved health are not synonymous. Weight reduction can be a marker of a changed lifestyle, but it can also be the result of a short-term restricted diet. It is confusing and misleading when the progress of a behavior change is measured by weight rather than by actual changes in behavior. This may promote an erroneous focus on lost pounds rather than on improved health.

A second problem is that if weight loss is the measure of success during the weight-loss phase, then how do we measure success during weight maintenance? Adjusting lifestyle choices to maintain weight and optimize health are lifelong challenges. Recording progress as successful changes in behavior reinforces the goal. By using a problem-solving model and by focusing on healthy behaviors instead of weight, the same educational model is used for weight reduction and weight maintenance. Patients will have been practicing the skills they need for weight maintenance long before they reach that stage. The problem-solving approach avoids the methodological gap between weight loss and weight maintenance.

This is not to suggest that people trying to lose weight should not be weighed. Weight changes let you know whether the behavior changes are effective. It provides feedback on the appropriateness of caloric intake. Sometimes people eat too little; other times they eat more than they realize. Weight is a reality check. However, there are many positive health changes that will not be detected by weight. Changes in blood pressure, lipid profiles, energy levels, and the fit of clothing also provide feedback.

Those successful at long-term weight maintenance report finding ways to

1. Continue engaging in high levels of physical activity (200–300 minutes per week and, for some, 1 hour a day)
2. Continue eating a diet lower in calories and fat (than intake before weight loss)

Helpful strategies to accomplish these were

1. Developing and maintaining consistent eating patterns
2. Eating breakfast
3. Regular self-monitoring of weight and/or eating behaviors
4. Watching less television
5. Acknowledging and addressing small "slips" before they become larger gains in weight

Based on Donnelly (2009), Wing (2005), and National Weight Control Registry (2011).

# Recognize the Difference between Hunger and Craving

Many patients are unable to distinguish between hunger and craving when they start a weight-reduction program. In the beginning of a weight-reduction period, patients were asked to describe hunger. They described it as uneasiness, a very uncomfortable feeling that one wanted to get rid of or avoid.

Being hungry may be justifiable and endured during a short period of weight loss. Decreasing numbers on the scale offer compensation for the hunger. During weight maintenance, when the intake of energy balances the expenditure, sensations of hunger may persist even though there is no need for additional calories. Appetite hormones may be in flux and psychological cues perceived as hunger.

It is during this time that cravings often become a problem that requires attention. If emotional eating and craving have not been addressed earlier in a weight-reduction program, they have to be tackled and dealt with during maintenance. Otherwise, they will jeopardize dietary management and sustained weight loss and maintenance.

# Prepare for Lapses and Relapses

A lapse is a temporary deviation from a behavior plan, and a relapse is a return to an old habit. Lapses are natural when anyone tries to maintain a behavior change, and it is the reason why maintenance needs to be included in all behavior change activities. The way patients manage lapse and relapse situations reveals much about how they will maintain newly acquired behaviors. Patients often experience disappointment, shame, and frustration from lapses and relapses. These feelings can keep them from contacting their health care providers for support. We can make a significant contribution to our lapsing and/or relapsing patients by encouraging them to consider their lapses and relapses as learning experiences. Try to help them remember and rediscover the motivation and goals that brought about the original changes in behavior. Lapses can contribute to the patient's increased understanding of the problem. A lapse could lead the patient to identify a new problem and to modify his or her plan. Perri (2001) found that weight maintainers trained in problem solving achieved better long-term weight-loss maintenance compared with weight maintainers solely trained in relapse prevention.

Some obese people are prone to black-or-white thinking, which interferes with viewing a lapse or relapse as a learning experience. Instead of asking themselves what went wrong or what could have been done to

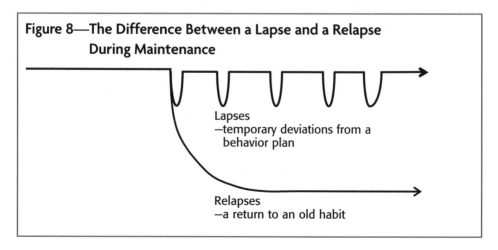

**Figure 8—The Difference Between a Lapse and a Relapse During Maintenance**

Lapses
—temporary deviations from a behavior plan

Relapses
—a return to an old habit

prevent relapses in the future, they may view themselves as failures or lay other extreme value judgments upon themselves. When a patient succeeds in returning to the plan after a lapse, his or her self-efficacy and motivation increase. Including a maintenance period to support and strengthen newly acquired habits helps prevent relapses and improves long-term results (Fig. 8) (Perri 2001).

Learning to recognize and prepare for situations that raise the possibility of lapses and/or relapses is a way to avoid them. Strategies for high-risk situations can be planned and practiced. If the patient has a very busy, stressful life, then the risks of a lapse are very high; therefore, we must be careful to not overlook the essential value of training our patients in lapse-prevention strategies.

---

### Help the Patient Uncover High-Risk Situations and Lapse-Prevention Strategies

Using open-ended sentences and restatement of personal goals can help patients identify high-risk situations and identify coping strategies or alternative solutions. Help patients structure their statements into open-ended statements like those below.
- "My goal right now is to..."
- "To reach this goal, I have to..."
- "I may face obstacles when..."
- "I will overcome these obstacles by..."
- "To keep my motivation, I will..."
- "I will reward myself by..."
- "I watch for signs that I am losing my motivation by..."
- "When I see one of these signs, I will turn to _____ or _____ for support."

---

# Encourage Support Systems

Social support can greatly assist patients in their efforts to maintain behavior change (Wing 2001, Wolfe 2004). Having sources of support helps people maintain and build on their positive lifestyle changes. Support may come from a spouse, a family member, different kinds of support groups, and health care personnel. National organizations and neighborhood communities can organize self-help groups that support behavior changes. Joining a self-help group is often a useful and inexpensive form of getting support. These groups tend to encourage long-term participation and are valuable complements to professional care. Many patients find support in weekly weigh-in appointments as a way of staying focused on their goals. Patients with access to the internet may find support by using online chat rooms, tracking systems, and mentoring programs (DMOZ 2011). Overall, patients are more likely to maintain progress if they use a support system, but they might require help identifying and developing support sources that work for them.

# Teach Self-Reward

Starting a new behavior is easier when there is a reward associated with the behavior. Patients benefit from learning to reward their behavior changes and to not base their lives on numbers on the scale. Helping patients learn how to reward themselves not only facilitates their implementation of the new behaviors, but also prepares the patients for rewarding (and thereby supporting) themselves during the maintenance period, when no weight loss is expected. Obese patients often use oral rewards. It can be a challenge for patients to plan personal rewards, and finding noneating methods of reward is often even more difficult. Obviously, what constitutes a reward will vary greatly between individuals. Look for rewards that will be special; something they would not routinely enjoy anyway.

Rewards might come at the end of the hour (no snacks), after a meal (ate as planned), after an activity (went grocery shopping), at the end of the day (no junk food), at the end of the week (accumulated three hours of physical activity), or at the end of the month (ate breakfast 20 out of 30 days). More frequent rewards are likely to be more helpful early in the behavior change process. Rewards can also be accumulated. For example, a patient could put a quarter in a jar as a short-term reward and spend the money when enough is accumulated to purchase something nice.

---

## Identifying Possible Rewards

After explaining the concept and rationale for providing self-rewards, ask questions like these.
- "How might you reward yourself for trying a new behavior?"
- "In what situations will you reward yourself?"
- "Would you like to learn how to reward yourself? What do you need and from whom?"
- "What rewards would you suggest for someone like yourself?"
- "How do you feel about rewarding yourself with something other than food?"
- "What rewards would fit within your budget?"
- "Is there anything you would like to reward yourself with but have not yet tried?"
- "Would you like some ideas?" (Here are some examples: buy flowers, go to a movie, get a massage, call a friend, buy a book, set aside 30 minutes a day to do whatever you want, get tickets to a ball game or concert, buy new clothes, etc. Putting an X on the calendar to indicate that a goal has been accomplished is sometimes enough reward for some people.)

---

# Reinforce Realism

## For Weight-Loss Goals

Weight maintenance may involve personal acceptance of a weight and body shape previously regarded as unacceptable (Foster 2005). Research shows that most people set weight-loss goals well beyond their reasonable reach and at levels much greater than those needed for health benefits.

A discrepancy between goal weight and actual weight loss can cause a halfhearted, "why-bother" attitude toward investment in weight maintenance. Some people who do accomplish their behavior goals and reduce their metabolic risk factors are still unhappy because they didn't reach their goal weight. After some discussion, they may be able to make peace with achieving less weight loss if they realize that they did meet the rationale for the original target (e.g., reduce risk factors), even if the target itself was not met (e.g., lose 30 pounds).

## For Life after Weight Loss

Patients often change their early expectations of living at a lower weight. Life after weight loss rarely matches the glamour portrayed in commercials for weight-loss programs. Even if Mrs. Doe enjoys wearing a smaller dress for her class reunion, day-to-day living—with all of its ups and downs—continues. As one patient told us, "It's not that I experience fewer problems being normal weight than I did being obese. There will always be problems and obstacles in life. But my attitude when they turn up has changed. Now I address the problems and do my best to solve them instead of denying them." Another patient describes her post–weight-loss experience like this: "I am sensitive to stress and am careful not to overbook my calendar, which I used to do. This was the main reason behind my excessive eating."

Emotional eating is one of the more persistent problems for people trying to maintain weight loss. Emotional eating disappears for some as they master the problem-solving process. Others look for coping strategies to avoid the consequences of emotional eating. One strategy is to join a support group in which the participants have an extensive forum to address and explore the feelings and problematic situations previously soothed by eating. Some find relief by discussing these topics with other people. Still others function as "restrained eaters," who develop strategies for keeping their meals structured and for curbing their cravings as a way of maintaining weight loss.

Lifestyle changes require lifelong attention. Problems do not end; they change. This behavioral approach to weight loss is a tool for life.

---

## Some Words to Remember about Behavioral Change

- It does not promise beauty, but it will improve your health.
- It is not a quick process, but slow and methodical.
- It is not easy, but often difficult and sometimes painful.
- It does not tell you what to do, but helps you decide what is worth doing.
- It does not take responsibility for your choices, but offers information and support so you can make informed choices.
- It is not prepackaged, but a custom-designed program for you by you.
- It does not apply external forces, but seeks to help you discover the forces within yourself.
- It does not judge your circumstances, but helps you live with them.
- It does not solve your problems, but offers tools to solve them.
- It does not simplify weight loss, but acknowledges its complexity.
- It is not an easy sell, but a path to real and lasting change.

---

# Appendix

## Meal Habits and Ideas for Change

### What and How Much I Eat over 24 Hours

*You will have a better idea of where you can make changes in your eating habits if you track them closely. Use this chart to record everything you eat and what you're doing while you eat for a 24-hour period.*

5 am _____

6 _____

7 _____

8 _____

9 _____

10 _____

11 _____

12 pm _____

1 _____

2 _____

3 _____

4 _____

5 _____

6 _____

| | |
|---|---|
| 7 | _____ |
| 8 | _____ |
| 9 | _____ |
| 10 | _____ |
| 11 | _____ |
| 12 am | _____ |
| 1 | _____ |
| 2 | _____ |
| 3 | _____ |
| 4 | _____ |

## Examine Your Record

*By looking closely at the record of what you eat and of your eating habits, you can have a better idea of what to do. Try answering these questions when you look at the record.*

Is anything missing in my diet? _____

Is there too much or too little of anything? _____

Are healthy snacks included? _____

Are the meals spread out over the day? _____

Did I eat breakfast? _____

## Usual Eating Schedule over 24 Hours

| | AM | | | | | | | | | | | | PM | | | | | | | | | | | | AM |
|---|---|---|---|---|---|---|---|---|---|---|---|---|---|---|---|---|---|---|---|---|---|---|---|---|---|---|
| | 5 | 6 | 7 | 8 | 9 | 10 | 11 | noon | 1 | 2 | 3 | 4 | 5 | 6 | 7 | 8 | 9 | 10 | 11 | mid-night | 1 | 2 | 3 | 4 | | |
| Food | | | | | | | | | | | | | | | | | | | | | | | | | | |
| Exercise | | | | | | | | | | | | | | | | | | | | | | | | | | |
| Sleep | | | | | | | | | | | | | | | | | | | | | | | | | | |

### KEY

*Place letters in the box representing the hour during which the activity occurred. For example, to record a snack eaten at 3:30 pm, place an "S" in the box under 3 pm.*

Food: Put M1, M2, and M3 in box for time of 1st, 2nd, and 3rd meals of the day
Put S in box for when a snack is eaten

Exercise: Put E in box for time of exercise

Sleep: Put X in all boxes representing when you were sleeping

*Look for pattterns that may help or hinder your goals.*

# Risky Situations

*Below are situations that can easily disrupt healthy routines. Mark the situations you think are most likely to interfere with your good habits.*

☐ Losing motivation

☐ Eating at a restaurant

☐ Eating at a buffet

☐ Feeling depressed

☐ Not having the "right" food available

☐ Holidays, like Christmas, Thanksgiving, etc.

☐ Difficulty saying no

☐ Not having a "Plan B"

☐ Lack of time for planning

☐ Eating too much on weekends

☐ Missing physical activity

☐ Being sick

☐ Other: _____

☐ Other: _____

# Reasons for Overeating

*Here are some reasons for unplanned eating and overeating. Place an X in each row to indicate how much each of these applies to you.*

| I overeat or have unplanned eating when... | Never | Seldom | Some-times | Often |
|---|---|---|---|---|
| • The food tastes and smells good | | | | |
| • I have a hard time saying no when food is offered | | | | |
| • I am eating with others | | | | |
| • It is a habit | | | | |
| • I feel low | | | | |
| • I am in pain | | | | |
| • I am stressed | | | | |
| • I feel lonely | | | | |
| • I am tired | | | | |
| • I am having difficulty sleeping | | | | |
| • I have anxiety or worries | | | | |
| • Other reason: | | | | |

# Resources

## Internet Weight-Loss Resources

Internet weight-loss programs can reach many people who do not have access to traditional treatment. However, tools are helpful only if they are used. Currently, users appear not to be optimally utilizing key aspects of available weight-loss interventions, such as education, monitoring, and support (Binks 2010).

**www.backontrackwithbarbara.com**
An internet mentoring program that offers memberships for 26 or 52 weeks.

**www.balancedweightmanagement.com**
Because there is no one answer to making the personal changes required for weight loss, this eclectic site provides information on multiple approaches from numerous authors.

**www.dmoz.org/Health/Weight_Loss/Support_Groups/**
**Chats_and_Forums/**
A list of online chats and forums.

**www.fitday.com**
Tools to plan and track weight loss, with records, reports, and food composition. Free.

**www.habitforge.com**

For those who need reminders, this free site offers an app that checks in daily. There is a blog, too.

**www.nwcr.ws**

Read success stories of people who have maintained weight loss at the National Weight Control Registry.

**www.sparkpeople.com**

Comprehensive free website offering calorie plans, fitness plans, recipes, motivation, tracking, and more.

**www.tcme.org**

The Center for Mindful Eating offers tips for paying attention to the eating process.

**http://win.niddk.nih.gov/index.htm**

The Weight-control Information Network (WIN) provides links to patient and professional resources.

# Nutrition Resources

**www.calorieking.com**

This website provides access to extensive nutrient composition information for single food items. To collect information for a whole meal, there is a charge. That charge also includes recommended calorie levels, tracking of food and exercise, and tips to support weight loss.

**http://choosemyplate.gov**

The U.S. Department of Agriculture's dietary guidelines and other reliable nutrition information.

**www.diabetes.org/food-and-fitness/food/my-food-advisor**
Track what you eat, find out nutrition information for thousands of foods, find healthy recipes, and count nutrients with the American Diabetes Association's MyFoodAdvisor online tool.

**www.dietaryguidelines.gov**
The 2010 *Dietary Guidelines for Americans* defines the US federal policy on nutrition and nutrition education.

**www.eatright.org**
Visit the website of the Academy of Nutrition and Dietetics for current information on weight management, diabetes, food safety, and a variety of other topics. Follow the link "Find a Registered Dietitian" to find one near you.

**www.fda.gov/ForConsumers/ConsumerUpdates/default.htm**
A consumer resource containing updates on the safety of dietary supplements and other products.

**www.nutrition.gov**
Nutrition.gov provides easy, online access to US government information on food and nutrition for consumers.

**http://ods.od.nih.gov/HealthInformation/makingdecisions.sec.aspx**
Learn about dietary supplements. The site opens to information for consumers but leads to more in-depth information for those interested.

# Obesity Education and Research

**www.obesity.org**

Learn more about obesity research and treatment from the Obesity Society.

**www.obesityaction.org**

The Obesity Action Coalition (OAC) is a nonprofit patient organization that provides education and advocates for those affected by obesity.

# Clinic Supplies

These three sites offer products specifically made for larger adults. (Sites may change, but others will take their place.)

**www.allegromedical.com/attr-condition-Obesity.html**

Medical supply site advertising devices to assist mobility, personal care, and comfort for larger adults.

**www.discountseniorsupply.com/category_pages/bariatric.asp**

Includes products designed for individuals weighing 250–700 pounds.

**www.fatcatalog.com**

Advertises a variety of commercial furniture and equipment but includes more specialized items, such as a wheelchair-accessible desk, oversized cardio equipment, and bariatric scales.

# Children's and Family Health

**www.ellynsatter.com**

A dietitian and social worker addresses the feeding relationship. Help with feeding a healthy family.

**www.letsmove.gov**

Let's Move! is a national program to encourage kids to eat healthy and move more.

**www.shapingamericasyouth.org/Default.aspx**

Provides multiple national and community links to resources and activities for healthy kids.

# Other Resources

*1,000 Years of Diabetes Wisdom: Inspiration and insight the world's leading diabetes professionals gained from their patients* by David Marrero, Robert Anderson, Martha Funnell, and Melinda Maryniuk (American Diabetes Association, 2008)

A glimpse of some ah-ha moments. Stories of how professionals learned from their patients and changed their approach to care in response.

**www.health.gov/paguidelines**

Physical Activity Guidelines for Americans describes the types and amounts of physical activity that offer substantial health benefits to Americans.

**www.healthfinder.gov**

An enormous database of health resources from over 1,600 government and nonprofit organizations, putting highly reliable information at your fingertips.

**http://ndep.nih.gov**

Are you at risk for diabetes? This site helps people determine their risk and offers ways to help prevent the disease.

**www.nhlbi.nih.gov/guidelines/obesity/bmi_tbl.htm**

Body mass index table.

# References

Adamson TE, Gullion DS: Assessment of diabetes continuing medical education. *Diabetes Care* 9:11–16, 1986

Adolfsson B, Carlson A, Undén AL, Rössner S: A qualitative evaluation of a behaviour modification weight reduction programme. *Health Educ J* 61:244–258, 2002

Adolfsson B, Elofsson S, Rössner S, Undén AL: Are sexual dissatisfaction and sexual abuse associated with obesity? A population based study. *Obes Res* 12:1702–1709, 2004

Al Harakeh AB, Burkhamer KJ, Kallies KJ, B, Mathiason MA, Kothari SN: Natural history and metabolic consequences of morbid obesity for patients denied coverage for bariatric surgery. *Surg Obes Relat Dis* 6:591–596, 2010

Anderson RM, Funnell MM: *The Art of Empowerment: Stories and Strategies for Diabetes Educators.* 2nd ed. Alexandria, VA, American Diabetes Association, 2005

Anderson RM, Funnell MM: Patient empowerment: myths and misconceptions. *Patient Educ Couns* 79:277–282, 2010

Anderson RM, Funnell MM, Aikens JE, Krein SL, Fitzgerald JT, Nwankwo R, Tannas CL, Tang TS: Evaluating the efficacy of an empowerment-based self-management consultant intervention: results of a two-year randomized controlled trial. *Ther Patient Educ* 1:3–11, 2009

Anderson RM, Funnell MM, Butler PM, Arnold MS, Fitzgerald JT, Feste CC: Patient empowerment: results from a randomized controlled trial. *Diabetes Care* 18:943–949, 1995

Astrup A, Finer N: Redefining type 2 diabetes: "diabesity" or "obesity dependent diabetes mellitus"? *Obes Rev* 1:57–59, 2000

Ayman B, Harakeh A, Burkhamer KJ, Kallies KJ, Mathiason MA, Kothari SN: Natural history and metabolic consequences of morbid obesity for patients denied coverage for bariatric surgery. *Surg Obes Relat Dis* 6:591–596, 2010

Bacon JC, Scheltema KE, Robinson BE: Fat phobia scale revised: the short form. *Int J Obes Relat Metab Disord* 25:252–257, 2001

Baker DW, Sudano JJ, Albert JM, Borawski EA, Dor A: Lack of health insurance and decline in overall health in late middle age. *N Engl J Med* 345:1106–1112, 2001

Bandura A: Self-efficacy: toward a unifying theory of behavioral change. *Psychol Rev* 84:191–215, 1977

Bandura A: Social cognitive theory: an agentic perspective. *Annu Rev Psychol* 52:1-26, 2001

Barkin SL, Heerman WJ, Warren MD, Rennhoff C: Millennials and the world of work: the impact of obesity on health and productivity. *J Bus Psychol* 25:239–245, 2010

Battersby M, Von Korff M, Schaefer J, Davis C, Ludman E, Greene SM, Parkerton M, Wagner EH: Twelve evidence-based principles for implementing self-management support in primary care. *Jt Comm J Qual Patient Saf* 36:561–570, 2010

Berkel LA, Poston WSC, Reeves RS, Foryet JP: Behavioral interventions for obesity. *J Am Diet Assoc* 105 (5 Suppl. 1):S35–S43, 2005

Binks M, van Mierlo T: Utilization patterns and user characteristics of an ad libitum internet weight loss program. *J Med Internet Res* 12:e9, 2010.

Björntorp P, Holm G, Rosmond R: Hypothalamic arousal, insulin resistance, and type 2 diabetes mellitus. *Diabet Med* 16:373–383, 1999

Blair SN: Physical activity: part A: overview. In *Managing Obesity: A Clinical Guide*. Foster GD, Nonas CA, Eds. Chicago, IL, American Dietetic Association, 2004, p. 119–128

Bob P, Fedor-Freybergh P, Jasova D, Bizik G, Susta M, Pavlat J, Zima T, Benakova H, Raboch J:   Dissociative symptoms and neuroendocrine dysregulation in depression. *Med Sci Monit* 14:499–504, 2008

Brownell K, Puhl K: Ways of coping with obesity stigma: review and conceptual analysis. *Eat Behav* 4:53–78, 2003

Bruch H: *Eating Disorders: Obesity, Anorexia Nervosa, and the Person Within.* New York, Basic Books, 1973

Bulik CM, Brownley KA, Shapiro JR: Diagnosis and management of binge eating disorder. *World Psychiatry* 6:142–148, 2007

Business Week Online: How safe are diet supplements? 30 Jan 2006. Accessed 17 Feb 2006. Available from http://www.businessweek.com/magazine/content/06_05/b3969068.htm

Byrne S, Cooper Z, Fairburn C: Weight maintenance and relapse in obesity: a qualitative study. *Int J Obes Relat Metab Disord* 27:955–962, 2003

Carlson A: *Reforming Diabetes Care in General Practice: Evaluation of Two Strategies for the Development of the Organisation and Quality of Health Care: The Department of Endocrinology, Karolinska Institutet, The Department of Psychology, Stockholm University, and the WHO*

*Collaborating Centre for Diabetes in Primary Care and Its Evaluation.* PhD thesis. Stockholm, Sweden, 1990

Carmichael MS, Humbert R, Dixen J, Palmisano G, Greenleaf W, Davidson JM: Plasma oxytocin increases in human sexual response. *J Clin Endocrinol Metab* 64:27–31, 1987

CDC: *Healthy weight—it's not a diet, it's a lifestyle!* Last updated: 15 Feb 2011[a]. Accessed 21 Mar 2011. Available from http://www.cdc.gov/healthyweight/physical_activity/index.html

CDC: *National Diabetes Fact Sheet: National estimates and general information on diabetes and prediabetes in the United States, 2011.* Atlanta, GA, U.S. Department of Health and Human Services, Centers for Disease Control and Prevention, 2011

CDC: *Overweight and obesity.* Last updated 21 Jun 2010. Accessed 14 Nov 2010. Available from http://www.cdc.gov/obesity/defining.html

CDC: *Physical Activity for Everyone.* Last updated 16 Feb 2011[b]. Assessed 21 Mar 2011. Available from http://www.cdc.gov/physicalactivity/everyone/guidelines/adults.html

CDC: Prevalence of disabilities and associated health conditions among adults—United States, 1999. *MMWR* 50:120–125, 2001. Last reviewed 2 May 2001. Accessed 21 Mar 2011. Available from http://www.cdc.gov/mmwr/preview/mmwrhtml/mm5007a3.htm

CDC, National Center for Health Statistics: *A Program for Early Release of Selected Estimates from the National Health Interview Survey.* Updated Sept 2011. Accessed 21 Sept 2011. Available from http://www.cdc.gov/nchs/nhis.htm

Chan JM, Rimm EB, Colditz GA, Stampfer MJ, Willett WC: Obesity, fat distribution, and weight gain as risk factors for clinical diabetes in men. *Diabetes Care* 17:961–969, 1994

Chaput JP, Klingenberg L, Sjödin A: Do all sedentary activities lead to weight gain: sleep does not. *Curr Opin Clin Nutr Metab Care* 13:601–607, 2010

Chilton M, Booth S: Hunger of the body and hunger of the mind: African American women's perceptions of food insecurity, health and violence. *J Nutr Educ Behav* 39:116–125, 2007

Colditz GA, Willett WC, Stampfer MJ, Manson JE, Hennekens CH, Arky RA, Speizer FE: Weight as a risk factor for clinical diabetes in women. *Am J Epidemiol* 132:501–513, 1990

Cooper P, Bowshill R: Dysphoric mood and overeating. *J Clin Psychol* 25:155–156, 1986

Cooper Z, Fairburn CG: A new cognitive behavioral approach to the treatment of obesity. *Behav Res Ther* 39:499–511, 2001

Cooper Z, Fairburn CG, Hawker DM: *Cognitive-Behavioral Treatment of Obesity*. New York, Guilford Press, 2003

Crossow NH, Jeffery RW, McGuire MT: Understanding weight stigmatization: A focus group study. *J Nutr Educ Behav* 33:208–214, 2001

Daly A, Michael P, Johnson EQ, Harrington CC, Patrick S, Bender T: Diabetes white paper: defining the delivery of nutrition services in Medicare medical nutrition therapy vs Medicare diabetes self-management training programs. *J Am Diet Assoc* 109:528–539, 2009

Dausch J: Determining when obesity is a disease. *J Am Diet Assoc* 101:293, 2001

Davis JL, Combs-Lane AM, Smith DW: Victimization and health risk behaviors: implications for prevention programs. In *Health Consequences of Abuse in the Family: A Clinical Guide for Evidence-Based Practice (Application and Practice in Health Psychology)*. Kendall-Tackett KA, Ed. Washington, DC, American Psychological Association, 2003, p. 179–195

De Ridder D: What is wrong with coping assessment? A review of conceptual and methodological issues. *Psychol Health* 12:417–431, 1997

DMOZ Open Directory Project. Accessed 28 Feb 2011. Available from http://www.dmoz.org/Health/Weight_Loss/Support_Groups/Chats_and_Forums/

Donnelly JE, Blair SN, Jakicic JM, Manore MM, Rankin JW, Smith BK: American College of Sports Medicine Position Stand: appropriate physical activity intervention strategies for weight loss and prevention of weight regain for adults. *Med Sci Sports Exerc* 41:459–471, 2009

Dowd J: Nutrition management after gastric bypass surgery. *Diabetes Spectrum* 18:82–84, 2005

Eckel RH, Grundy SM, Zimmet PZ: The metabolic syndrome. *Lancet* 365:1415–1428, 2005

Englehard C, Garson A, Dorn S. *Reducing Obesity: Policy Strategies from the Tobacco Wars.* The Urban Institute. Updated Jul 2009. Available from http://www.urban.org/publications/411926.html

Fabricatore AN, Wadden TA, Womble LG, Sarwer DB, Berkowitz RI, Foster GD, Brock JR: The role of patients' expectations and goals in the behavioral and pharmacological treatment of obesity. *Int J Obes* 31:1739–1745, 2007

FDA (2010[b]): *FDA Drug Safety Communication: FDA Recommends Against the Continued Use of Meridia (sibutramine).* Last updated 10 Dec 2010. Accessed 3 Jan 2011. Available from http://www.fda.gov/Drugs/DrugSafety/ucm228746.htm

FDA: *FDA expands use of banding system for weight loss.* Last updated 16 Feb 2011. Accessed 13 Sept 2011. Available from http://www.fda.gov/NewsEvents/Newsroom/PressAnnouncements/ucm245617.htm

FDA: *FDA warns consumers not to use Fruta Planta weight loss products.* Last updated 3 Jan 2011[a]. Accessed 21 Mar 2011. Available from http://www.fda.gov/NewsEvents/Newsroom/PressAnnouncements/ucm238491.htm

FDA (2010[a]): *Orlistat (marketed as Alli and Xenical): Labeling Change.* Last updated 26 May 2010. Accessed 3 Jan 2011. Available from http://www.fda.gov/Safety/MedWatch/SafetyInformation/SafetyAlertsforHumanMedicalProducts/ucm213448.htm

FDAnews Drug Daily Bulletin: *FDA Declines to Approve Orexigen's Contrave, Requests New Trial.* Last updated 3 Feb 2011[b]. Accessed 26 Mar 2011. Available from http://www.fdanews.com/newsletter/article?articleId=133950&issueId=14435

Feldman M, Meyer I: Childhood abuse and eating disorders in gay and bisexual men. *Int J Eat Disord* 40:418–423, 2007

Fenkelstein EA, Dibonaventura M daCosta, Burgess SM, Hale BC: The costs of obesity in the workplace. *J Occup Environ Med* 52:971–976, 2010

Ferraro KF, Thorpe RJ Jr, Wilkinson JA: The life course of severe obesity: does childhood overweight matter? *J Gerontol B Psychol Sci Soc Sci* 58 (Suppl. 2):S110–S119, 2003

Feste C: A practical look at patient empowerment. *Diabetes Care* 15:922–925, 1992

Flicker L, McCaul KA, Hankey GJ, Jamrozik K, Brown WJ, Byles JE, Almeida OP: Body mass index and survival in men and women aged 70 to 75. *J Am Geriatr Soc* 58:234–241, 2010

Fontaine KR, Bartlett SJ: Commentary: access and use of medical care among obese persons. *Obes Res* 8:403–406, 2000

Foreyt JP, Goodrick GK: Attributes of successful approaches to weight loss and control. *Appl Prev Psychol* 3:209–215, 1995

Foster GD, Makris A: Behavioral treatment: part B: practical applications. In *Managing Obesity: A Clinical Guide*. Foster GD, Nonas CA, Eds. Chicago, IL, American Dietetic Association, 2004, p. 76–90

Foster GD, Makris AP, Bailer BA: Behavioral treatment of obesity. *Am J Clin Nutr* 82 (Suppl.):230S–235S, 2005

Franz MJ, VanWormer JJ, Crain AL, Boucher JL, Histon T, Caplan W, Bowman JD, Pronk NP: Weight-loss outcomes: a systematic review and meta-analysis of weight-loss clinical trials with a minimum 1-year follow-up. *J Am Diet Assoc* 107:1755–1767, 2007

Freud A: *The Ego and the Mechanisms of Defense*. London, Hogarth, 1979

Friedman KE, Reichmann SK, Costanzo PR, Zelli A, Ashmore JA, Musante GJ: Weight stigmatization and ideological beliefs: relation to psychological functioning in obese adults. *Obes Res* 13:907–913, 2005

Funnell MM, Anderson RM: Empowerment and self-management of diabetes. *Clinical Diabetes* 22:123–127, 2004

Glasglow RE, Orleans CT, Wagner EH, Curry SJ, Solberg LI: Does the chronic care model serve also as a template for improving prevention? *Milbank Quarterly* 79:579–612, 2001

Gooley J, Levich B: *"The Paradigm's a-'Changing:" Patient-centered approaches to behavior change.* Presented at the American Association of Diabetes Educators 32nd Annual Meeting and Exhibition, Washington, DC, 12 Aug 2005

Green Pastors JG, Arnold MS, Daly A, Franz M, Warshaw HS: *Diabetes Nutrition Q & A for Health Professionals*. Alexandria, VA, American Diabetes Association, 2003

Grumbach K, Bodenheimer T: Can health care teams improve primary care practice? *JAMA* 291:1246–1251, 2004

Grundy SM, Cleeman JI, Daniels SR, Donato KA, Eckel RH, Franklin BA, Gordon DJ, Krauss RM, Savage PJ, Smith SC Jr, Spertus JA, Costa F: Diagnosis and management of the metabolic syndrome: an American Heart Association/National Heart, Lung, and Blood Institute Scientific Statement: Executive Summary. *Circulation* 112:e285–e290, 2005

Henry JP, Stephens PM: *Stress, Health, and the Social Environment: A Sociobiologic Approach to Medicine.* New York, Springer-Verlag, 1977

Hill JO: Understanding and addressing the epidemic of obesity: an energy balance perspective. *Endocr Rev* 27:750–761, 2006

Hill JO, Thompson H, Wyatt H: Weight maintenance: what's missing? *J Am Diet Assoc* 105 (5 Suppl. 1):S63–S66, 2005

Hroscikoski MC, Solberg LI, Sper-Hillen JM, Harper PG, McGrail MP, Crabtree BF: Challenges of change: a qualitative study of chronic care model implementation. *Ann Fam Med* 4:317–326, 2006

Hörchner R, Tuinebreijer W, Kelder H, Urk E: Coping behavior and loneliness among obese patients *Obes Surg* 12:864–868, 2002

IDF: *The High Risk Approach.* Last updated 2010. Accessed 26 Dec 2010. Available from http://www.idf.org/diabetes-prevention/high-risk-approach

IDF: *The IDF Consensus Worldwide Definition of the Metabolic Syndrome.* Accessed 21 Mar 2011. Available from http://www.idf.org/metabolic-syndrome

International Association for the Study of Obesity: The Stock Conference March 2002: how much physical activity is enough to prevent unhealthy weight gain? *IASO Newsletter* 4:14–15, 2002

Ivy AS, Rex CS, Chen Y, Dubé C, Maras PM, Grigoriadis DE, Gall CM, Lynch G, Baram TZ: Hippocampal dysfunction and cognitive impairments provoked by chronic early-life stress involve excessive activation of CRH receptors. *J Neurosci* 30:13005–13015, 2010

Jastran M, Bisognib CA, Sobalc J, Blaked C, Devine CM: Eating routines: Embedded, value based, modifiable, and reflective. *Appetite* 52:127–136, 2009

Jeffery R, Rick A: Cross-sectional and longitudinal associations between body mass index and marriage-related factors. *Obes Res* 10:809–815, 2002

Kahn R, Buse J, Ferrannini E, Stern M: The metabolic syndrome: time for a critical appraisal: joint statement from the American Diabetes Association and the European Association for the Study of Diabetes. *Diabetes Care* 28:2289–2304, 2005

Kegan R: *In Over Our Heads: The Mental Demands of Modern Life.* Cambridge, MA, Harvard University Press, 1994

King TK, Clark MM, Pera V: History of sexual abuse and obesity treatment outcome. *Addict Behav* 21:283–290, 1996

Kjellström S: *Ansvar, Hälsa Och Makt* [in Swedish]. PhD thesis. Department of Health and Society, Linköping University, Sweden, 2005

Knowler WC, Barrett-Connor E, Fowler SE, Hamman RF, Lachin JM, Walker EA, Nathan DM, Diabetes Prevention Program Research Group: Reduction in the incidence of type 2 diabetes with lifestyle intervention or metformin. *N Engl J Med* 346:393–403, 2002

Kolotkin RL, Crosby RD, Williams GR: Health-related quality of life varies among obese subgroups. *Obes Res* 10:748–756, 2002

Korner J, Aronne LJ: The emerging science of body weight regulation and its impact on obesity treatment. *J Clin Invest* 11:565–570, 2003

Kulick D, Hark L, Deen D: The bariatric surgery patient: a growing role for registered dietitians. *J Am Diet Assoc* 110:593–599, 2010

Kushner RF, Blatner DJ: Risk assessment of the overweight and obese patient. *J Am Diet Assoc* 105 (5 Suppl. 1):S53–S62, 2005

Laitinen J, Ek E, Sovio U: Stress-related eating and drinking behavior and body mass index and predictors of this behavior. *Prev Med* 34:29–39, 2002

Larsson U, Karlsson J, Sullivan M: Impact of overweight and obesity on health-related quality of life—a Swedish population study. *Int J Obes Relat Metab Disord* 26:417–424, 2002

Lating JM, O'Reilly MA, Anderson KP: Eating disorders and posttraumatic stress: phenomenological and treatment considerations using the two-factor model. *Int J Emerg Ment Health* 4:113–118, 2002

Lazarus RS, Folkman S: *Stress, Appraisal and Coping*. New York, Springer, 1984

Lee CD, Blair SN, Jackson AS: Cardiorespiratory fitness, body composition, and all-cause and cardiovascular disease mortality in men. *Am J Clin Nutr* 69:373–380, 1999

Lee JS, Sheer JLO, Lopez N, Rosenbaum S: Coverage of obesity treatment: a state-by-state analysis of Medicaid and state insurance laws. *Public Health Rep* 125:596–604, 2010

Lemmens K, Stratin M, Huijsman R, Nieboer A: Professional commitment to changing chronic illness care: results from disease management programmes. *Int J Qual Health Care* 21:233–242, 2009

Lewin K: Action research and minority problems. *J Soc Issues* 34–46, Nov 1947

Link B, Phelan J: Conceptualizing stigma. *Annu Rev Sociol* 27:363–385, 2001

Ljung T: *Stress System Function in Abdominal Obesity: The Hypothalamic-Pituitary-Adrenal Axis and the Sympathetic Nervous System in Middle-Aged*

*Men*. PhD thesis. The Cardiovascular Institute, Gothenburg University, Sweden, 2001

Longitudinal Assessment of Bariatric Surgery (LABS) Consortium: Perioperative safety in the longitudinal assessment of bariatric surgery. *N Engl J Med* 361:445–454, 2009

Look AHEAD Research Group, Wing RR: Long-term effects of a lifestyle intervention on weight and cardiovascular risk factors in individuals with type 2 diabetes mellitus: four-year results of the Look AHEAD trial. *Arch Intern Med* 170:1566–1575, 2010

Lyon HN, Hirschhorn JN: Genetics of common forms of obesity: a brief overview. *Am J Clin Nutr* 82 (1 Suppl.):215S–217S, 2005

Maffeis C: Aetiology of overweight and obesity in children and adolescents. *Eur J Pediatr* 159 (Suppl. 1):S35–S44, 2000

Marcus DA: Obesity and the impact of chronic pain. *Clin J Pain* 20:186–191, 2004

Marshall JR, Neill J: The removal of a psychosomatic symptom: effects on the marriage. *Fam Process* 16:273–280, 1977

Maslow A: *Toward a Psychology of Being*. 2nd ed. Princeton, NJ, Van Nostrand, 1968

Mayer-Davis EJ, Bell RA, Dabelea D, D'Agostino R Jr, Imperatore G, Lawrence JM, Liu L, Marcovina S,.SEARCH for Diabetes in Youth Study Group: The many faces of diabetes in American youth: type 1 and type 2 diabetes in five race and ethnic populations: the SEARCH for Diabetes in Youth Study. *Diabetes Care* 32 (Suppl. 2):S99–S101, 2009

McDougall J: *Theatres of the Body*. London, Norton, 1989

McGuire MT, Wing RR, Hill JO: The prevalence of weight loss maintenance among American adults. *Int J Obes Relat Metab Disord* 23:1314–1319, 1999

Miller WR, Rollnick S: Facilitating change. In *Motivational Interviewing: Preparing People for Change.* 2nd ed. Miller WR, Rollnick S, Eds. New York, Guildford Press, 2002, p. 20–29

Mills JK: The obese personality: defense, compromise, symbiotic arrest, and the characterologically depressed self. *Issues in Psychoanalytic Psychology* 16:67–80, 1994

NAASO: National nutrition summit position paper. Accessed 16 Feb 2006. Available from http://www.obesity.org/publications/national-nutrition-summit-position-paper.htm

National Restaurant Association: *Facts at a Glance,* 2010. Accessed 29 Jan 2011. Available from http://www.restaurant.org/research

National Weight Control Registry: *NWCR facts.* Accessed 27 Sept 2011. Available from http://www.nwcr.ws/Research/default.htm

NCBI, National Institutes of Health, National Heart, Lung and Blood Institute: Clinical guidelines on the identification, evaluation and treatment of overweight and obesity in adults: the evidence report. Sept 1998. Accessed 2 Jan 2011. Available from http://www.ncbi.nlm.nih.gov/books/bookres.fcgi/obesity/obesity.pdf

NICE, National Institute for Health and Clinical Excellence: *Obesity: the prevention, identification, assessment and management of overweight and obesity in adults and children.* Dec 2006. Accessed 2 Jan 2011. Available from http://www.nice.org.uk/CG43

NHLBI: *Aim for a Healthy Weight,* 2005 (NIH Publication No. 05-5213). Accessed 13 Sept 2011. Available from http://www.nhlbi.nih.gov/health/public/heart/obesity/lose_wt/calories.htm

NHLBI: *Clinical Guidelines on the Identification, Evaluation, and Treatment of Overweight and Obesity in Adults: The Evidence Report..* Bethesda, MD, National Institutes of Health, 1998 (NIH publ. no. 98-4083). Accessed

21 Mar 2005. Available from http://www.nhlbi.nih.gov/guidelines/ obesity/ob_gdlns.htm

NHLBI: *The Practical Guide: Identification, Evaluation, and Treatment of Overweight and Obesity in Adults*. Bethesda, MD, National Institutes of Health, 2000 (NIH publ. no. 00-4084). Last accessed 6 Sept 2011. Available from www.nhlbi.nih.gov/guidelines/obesity/prctgd_c.pdf

NIDDK: *Prescription Medications for the Treatment of Obesity*. NIH publ. no. 07-4191. Updated 2007.

NIDDK, Weight-control Information Network: *Bariatric Surgery for Severe Obesity*. NIH publ. no. 08-4006. Updated Mar 2009. Accessed 2 Jan 2011. Available from http://win.niddk.nih.gov/publications/gastric. htm

NIH: *Diabetes Prevention Program (DPP)*.NIH publ. no. 09–5099. Updated Oct 2008. Accessed 27 Sept 2011. Available from http://diabetes.niddk. nih.gov/dm/pubs/preventionprogram

NIH Technology Assessment Conference Panel: Methods for voluntary weight loss and control. *Ann Intern Med* 116:942–949, 1992

Nonas CA, Foster GD: Obesity: an overview. In *Managing Obesity: A Clinical Guide*. Foster GD, Nonas CA, Eds. Chicago, IL, American Dietetic Association, 2004, p. 5–11

Ode JJ, Pivarnik JM, Reeves MJ, Knous JL: Body mass index as a predictor of percent fat in college athletes and nonathletes. *Med Sci Sports Exerc* 39:403–409, 2007

Ogden CL, Carroll MD: Prevalence of overweight, obesity, and extreme obesity among adults: United States, trends 1960–1962 through 2007–2008. NCHS Health E-Stats, CDC, National Center for Health Statistics. Last updated 6 June 2011. Accessed 18 Oct 2011. Available from http://www.cdc.gov/nchs/data/hestat/obesity_adult_07_08/ obesity_adult_07_08.htm

Papero D: *Bowen Family Systems Theory*. Needham Heights, MA, Allyn & Bacon, 1990

Patel SR, Redline S: Two epidemics: are we getting fatter as we sleep less? *Sleep* 27:602–603, 2004

Perri MG, Nezu AM, McKelvey WF, Shermer RL, Renjilian DA, Viegener BJ: Relapse prevention training and problem-solving therapy in the long-term management of obesity. *J Consult Clin Psychol* 69:722–726, 2001

Phillips A, Carroll D, Gale C, Lord J, Arlt W, Batty G: Cortisol, DHEAS, their ratio and the metabolic syndrome: evidence from the Vietnam Experience Study. *Eur J Endocrinol* 162:919–923, 2010

Pi-Sunyer FX: The epidemiology of central fat distribution in relation to disease. *Nutr Rev* 62:120–126, 2004

Pi-Sunyer X, Kris-Etherton PM: Improving health outcomes: future directions in the field. *J Am Diet Assoc* 105 (5 Suppl. 1):S14–S16, 2005

Picot J, Jones J, Colquitt JL, Gospodarevskaya E, Loveman E, Baxter L, Clegg AJ: The clinical effectiveness and cost-effectiveness of bariatric (weight loss) surgery for obesity: a systematic review and economic evaluation. *Health Technol Assess* 13:1–190, 215–357, iii–iv, 2009

Pollack A: FDA rejects Qnexa, a third weight-loss drug. *New York Times*, 29 Oct 2010[a]. Accessed 3 Jan 2011. Available from http://www.nytimes.com/2010/10/29/health/policy/29drug.html

Pollack A: No F.D.A. approval for new diet pill. *New York Times*, 23 Oct 2010. Accessed 26 Mar 2011. Available from http://www.nytimes.com/2010/10/24/business/24obesity.html

Popkess-Vawter S, Wendel S, Schmoll S, O'Connell K: Overeating, reversal theory, and weight cycling. *West J Nurs Res* 20:67–83, 1998

Porter JS, Bean MK, Gerke CK, Stern M: Psychosocial factors and
perspectives on weight gain and barriers to weight loss among
adolescents enrolled in obesity treatment. *J Clin Psychol Med Settings*
17:98–102, 2010

Poston WS 2nd, Foreyt JP: Successful management of the obese patient.
*Am Fam Physician* 61:3615–3622, 2000

Pritchett AM, Foreyt JP, Mann DL: Treatment of the metabolic
syndrome: the impact of lifestyle modification. *Curr Atheroscler Rep*
7:95–102, 2005

Prochaska JO, Norcross JC, DiClemente CC: *Changing for Good*. New
York, Avon Books, 1995

Puhl R, Brownell K: Ways of coping with obesity stigma: review and
conceptual analysis. *Eat Behav* 4:53–78, 2003

Puhl R, Heuer C: The stigma of obesity: a review and update. *Obesity*
17:941–964, 2009

Risérus U, Arnlöv J, Brismar K, Zethelius B, Berglund L, Vessby B:
Sagittal abdominal diameter is a strong anthropometric marker of
insulin resistance and hyperproinsulinemia in obese men. *Diabetes Care*
27:2041–2046, 2004

Risérus U, de Faire U, Berglund L, Hellénius ML: Sagittal abdominal
diameter as a screening tool in clinical research: cutoffs for
cardiometabolic risk. *J Obes* 2010. pii: 757939. Epub 11 Mar 2010

Robinson BE, Bacon JG: The 'If I only were thin…' treatment program:
decreasing the stigmatizing effects of fatness. *Prof Psychol Res Pr* 27:175–
183, 1996

Rock CL, Flatt SW, Sherwood NE, Karanja N, Pakiz B, Thomson CA:
Effect of a free prepared meal and incentivized weight loss program

on weight loss and weight loss maintenance in obese and overweight women: a randomized controlled trial. *JAMA* 304:1803–1810, 2010

Rogge MM, Greenwald M, Golden A: Obesity, stigma and civilized oppression. *ANS Adv Nurs Sci* 27:301–315, 2004

Rollnick S, Mason P, Butler C: *Health Behaviour Change: A Guide for Practitioners*. Edinburgh, U.K., Churchill Livingstone, 1999

Rosenstock IM, Strecher VJ, Becker MH: Social learning theory and the Health Belief Model. *Health Educ Q* 15:175–183, 1988

Rydén A: *Coping and Personality in the Obese: Results from the Swedish Obese Subjects Study*. PhD thesis. Department of Body Composition and Metabolism, Institute of Internal Medicine, Göteborg University, Göteborg, Sweden, 2003

Rydén O: In defense of obesity. In *Defense Mechanisms: Theoretical, Research, and Clinical Perspectives*. Hentschel U, Smith GJW, Draguns JG, Ehlers W, Eds. Amsterdam, Elsevier, 2004, p. 557–579

Sacks FM, Bray GA, Carey VJ, Smith SR, Ryan DH, Anton SD, McManus K, Champagne CM, Bishop LM, Laranjo N, Leboff MS, Rood JC, de Jonge L, Greenway FL, Loria CM, Obarzanek E, Williamson DA: Comparison of weight-loss diets with different compositions of fat, protein, and carbohydrates. *N Engl J Med* 360:859–873, 2009

Sapolsky RM: Why stress is bad for your brain. *Science* 273:749–750, 1996

Sarlio-Lähteenkorva S: Relapse stories in obesity. *Eur J Public Health* 8:203–209, 1998

Seidell JC: Waist circumference and waist/hip ratio in relation to all-cause mortality, cancer and sleep apnea. *Eur J Clin Nutr* 64:35–41, 2010

SIGN (Scottish Intercollegiate Guidelines Network): *Management of Obesity: A national clinical guideline* (publ. no. 115). Accessed 2 Jan 2011.

Available from http://www.sign.ac.uk/guidelines/fulltext/115/index. html

Slochower J, Kaplan SP: Anxiety, perceived control, and eating in obese and normal weight persons. *Appetite* 1:75–83, 1980

Slochower J, Kaplan SP, Mann L: The effects of life stress and weight on mood and eating. *Appetite* 2:115–125, 1981

Stegemann L: *Treating Weight Regain after Weight-Loss Surgery.* Last updated 4 Jan 2011. Accessed 22 Feb 2011. Available from http://www. obesityaction.org/magazine/oacnews8/healthqanda.php

Stern JS, Kazaks A, Downey M: Future and implications of reimbursement for obesity treatment. *J Am Diet Assoc* 105 (5 Suppl. 1):S104–S109, 2005

Stoeckle JD: The practice of primary care. In *Primary Care Medicine Office evaluation and management of the adult patient.* Sixth ed. Goroll AH, Mulley AG, Eds. Lipincott Williams & Wilkins, PA, 2009, p. 1–9

Strecher VJ, DeVellis BM, Becker MH, Rosenstock IM: The role of self-efficacy in achieving health behavior change. *Health Educ Q* 13:73–92, 1986

Stroebel CK, McDaniel RR Jr, Crabtree BF, Miller WL, Nutting PA, Stange KC: How complexity science can inform a reflective process for improvement in primary care practices. *Jt Comm J Qual Patient Saf* 31:438–446, 2005

Stuifbergen AK, Becker HA: Predictors of health-promoting lifestyles in persons with disabilities. *Res Nurs Health* 17:3–13, 1994

Teixeira ME, Budd GM: Obesity stigma: a newly recognized barrier to comprehensive and effective type 2 diabetes management. *J Am Acad Nurse Pract* 22:527–533, 2010

Top Achievement: *Creating S.M.A.R.T. goals.* Accessed 18 Oct 2011. Available from http://topachievement.com/smart.html

Tuomilehto J, Lindstrom J, Eriksson JG, Valle TT, Hamalainen H, Ilanne-Parikka P, Keinanen-Kiukaanniemi S, Laakso M, Louheranta A, Rastas M, Salminen V, Uusitupa M, Finnish Diabetes Prevention Study Group: Prevention of type 2 diabetes mellitus by changes in lifestyle among subjects with impaired glucose tolerance. *N Engl J Med* 344:1343–1350, 2001

U.S. Department of Agriculture, U.S. Department of Health and Human Services: *Dietary Guidelines for Americans, 2010.* 7th ed. Washington, DC, U.S. Govt. Printing Office, 2010. Accessed 20 Sept 2011. Available from *http://health.gov/dietaryguidelines/dga2010/dietaryguidelines2010. pdf*

U.S. Department of Health and Human Services: *2008 Physical Activity Guidelines for Americans.* Accessed 13 Sept 2011. Available from http://www.health.gov/PAGuidelines

U.S. Department of Health and Human Services: *America's Health Literacy: Why We Need Accessible Health Information. Accessed 27 Sept 2011.* Available from *www.health.gov/communication/literacy/issuebrief*

Uuvnäs-Moberg K, Bjorkstrand E, Hillegaart V, Ahlenius S: Oxytocin as a possible mediator of SSRI-induced antidepressant effects. *Psychopharmacology* 142:95–101, 1999

Vardar E, Caliyurt O, Arikan E, Tuglu C: Sleep quality and psychopathological features in obese binge eaters. *Stress Health* 20:35–41, 2004

Wagner EH, Austin BT, Davis C, Hindmarsh M, Schaefer J, Bonomi A: Improving chronic illness care: translating evidence into action. *Health Affairs* 20:64–89, 2001

Weight-control Information Network: *Overweight and Obesity Statistics.* Last updated Feb 2010. Accessed 6 Dec 2010. Available from http://win.niddk.nih.gov/statistics/index.htm

Wells AS, Read NW, Macdonald IA: Effects of carbohydrate and lipid on resting energy expenditure, heart rate, sleepiness, and mood. *Physiol Behav* 63:621–628, 1998

White S, Bissell P, Anderson C: A qualitative study of cardiac rehabilitation patients' perspectives on making dietary changes. *J Hum Nutr Diet* 24:122–127, 2011

WHO: BMI classification. Last updated 20 Mar 2011. Accessed 20 Mar 2011. Available from http://apps.who.int/bmi/index.jsp?introPage=intro_3.html

WHO: *Global Database on Body Mass Index.* Accessed 14 Sept 2011. Available from http://apps.who.int/bmi/index.jsp

WHO: *Global Recommendations on Physical Activity for Health.* Geneva, Switzerland, World Health Org., 2010[b]

WHO: *Obesity: Preventing and Managing the Global Epidemic: Report of a WHO Consultation on Obesity.* Geneva, World Health Org., 2000

WHO: *Obesity and Overweight.* Geneva, Switzerland, World Health Org., 2009

WHO: *WHO Expert Consultation on Waist Circumference and Waist-Hip Ratio.* Last updated 8–11 Dec 2008. Accessed 16 Jan 2011. Available from http://www.who.int/nutrition/topics/expert_consultation_wc_whr/en/

WHO Europe: *The Challenge of Obesity in the WHO European Region and the Strategies for Response.* Denmark, World Health Org., 2007. (ebook) ISBN 978928901409. Available from http://www.euro.who.int/__data/assets/pdf_file/0010/74746/E90711.pdf

Wiederman MW, Sansone RA, Sansone LA: Obesity among sexually abused women: an adaptive function for some? *Women Health* 29:89–100, 1999

Wilson B: Your eating habits inventory. Accessed 27 Sept 2011. Available from http://www.balancedweightmanagement.com/Your%20 Eating%20Habits%20Inventory.htm

Wilson C: *I'm Still Hungry: Finding Myself Through Thick and Thin.* Carlsbad, CA, Hay House, 2003

Wing RR, Hill JO: Successful weight loss maintenance. *Annu Rev Nutr* 21:323–341, 2001

Wing RR, Phelan S: Long-term weight loss maintenance. *Am J Clin Nutr* 82(1 Suppl.):222S–225S, 2005

Wolfe WA: A review: maximizing social support – a neglected strategy for improving weight management with African-American women. *Ethn Dis* 14:212–218, 2004

Zgibor JC, Peyrot M, Ruppert K, Noullet W, Siminerio LM, Peeples M, McWilliams J, Koshinsky J, DeJesus C, Emerson S, Charron-Prochownik D, AADE/UPMC Diabetes Education Outcomes Project: Using the American Association of Diabetes Educators Outcomes System to identify patient behavior change goals and diabetes educator responses. *Diabetes Educ* 33:839–842, 2007

Zhao J, Bradfield JP, Li M, Wang K, Zhang H, Kim CE, Annaiah K, Glessner JT, Thomas K, Garris M, Frackelton EC, Otieno FG, Shaner JL, Smith RM, Chiavacci RM, Berkowitz RI, Hakonarson H, Grant SF: The role of obesity-associated loci identified in genome-wide association studies in the determination of pediatric BMI. *Obesity* 17:2254–2257, 2009

Zhao J, Grant SF: Genetics of childhood obesity. *J Obes* 2011:845148, Epub 26 May 2011

Zimmet P, Alberti KG, Shaw J: Global and societal implications of the diabetes epidemic. *Nature* 414:782–787, 2001

Zinn A: Unconventional wisdom about the obesity epidemic *Am J Med Sci* 340:481–491, 2010

Zwarenstein M, Goldman J, Reeves S: Interprofessional collaboration: effects of practice-based interventions on professional practice and healthcare outcomes. *Cochrane Database System Rev* no. CD000072, 2009

# Index